The Weight of Scrubs: Nurses and the Trauma of Violence

Shireen

First Printing, 2024

Table of Contents

CHAPTER 1. INTRODUCTION

The healthcare industry leads all other sectors in the incidence of nonfatal workplace assaults (Emergency Nurses Association, 2023). Researchers suggested the detrimental impact workplace violence (WPV) has on nurses in the healthcare setting (Báez-León et al., 2016; Beattie et al., 2019; Bildik et al., 2022; Dadashzadeh et al., 2019; Doehring et al., 2023; Kiymaz & Koç, 2023; Lim et al., 2022; Moman et al., 2020; Nevels et al., 2020; Ogboghodo & Okojie, 2020). Lim et al. (2022) mentioned that violence compromises the quality of patient care delivery for these nurses' communities. This researcher designed this small exploratory master's thesis research study to utilize a qualitative research methodology using Husserl and Heidegger's phenomenology approach to ask open-ended questions in semi-structured interviews that explored the lived experiences of nurses and their encounters with WPV and how this affects their role as a nurse (Polit & Beck, 2021).

Background of the Study

Lim et al. (2022) stated that nurses frequently have the most patient interaction, leaving them as an easy target for frustration and violence. The Occupational Safety and Health Administration (OSHA) defines *WPV* as any harassment, intimidation, or verbal abuse, ranging from threats of physical violence to homicide (OSHA, n.d.). Lim et al. also discussed that psychological violence, a form of WPV, is the intent to use power to threaten another individual by impairing physical, mental, spiritual, moral, or social health. Lim et al. advised that harassment, such as insults, bullying, and intimidation, are additional forms of WPV.

Moman et al. (2020) revealed that in a study conducted by the United States Veterans Health Administration, through distributing surveys at a pain management conference, providers reported that 41% of assaults on healthcare workers occur in inpatient psychiatric units, yet 59% of assaults occur elsewhere within healthcare institutions. Kiymaz and Koç (2023) used a mixed-methods study to research WPV among emergency department (ED) nurses and how WPV correlated to occupational commitment and intention to resign. Kiymaz and Koç determined that emotional commitment to the nursing profession might decrease, and nurses' intention to resign may rise as exposure to aggression and violence increases.

This researcher studied the phenomenon of WPV among nurses because there has been an extensive variation in the effectiveness of the current healthcare policies to mitigate violence. Using Ida Jean Orlando's nursing process discipline theory, nurses must utilize their perceptions and feelings to guide them through a patient's distress and violent behaviors to examine their immediate needs and de-escalate violent behaviors (Orlando, 1961, as cited in Petiprin, 2023). WPV in healthcare is a global problem, and this researcher sought a unique perspective on the experiences of violence to approach the issue with new potential solutions.

Need for the Study

While research has been ongoing to examine WPV in healthcare, evidence from current researchers suggested that data-driven solutions are still needed to resolve this healthcare epidemic (Báez-León et al., 2016; Beattie et al., 2019; Bildik et al.,

2022; Dadashzadeh et al., 2019 Doehring et al., 2023; Kiymaz & Koç, 2023; Lim et al., 2022; Moman et al., 2020; Nevels et al., 2020; Ogboghodo & Okojie, 2020). This researcher designed this study to target gaps in the existing literature by investigating the experience of WPV against nurses from a different perspective. This researcher's data emphasized factors that led to violence in healthcare, considerations that assisted the WPV education planning for nurses, influences that improved WPV policy reform, and the support nurses received from the nursing administration after WPV had occurred. This researcher's data generated solutions to decrease the likelihood of nurses leaving the healthcare industry by understanding the nurses' perspective of WPV in healthcare.

Purpose of the Study

The Joint Commission (TJC) has emphasized the need to resolve WPV in healthcare settings, implementing new regulatory standards of WPV prevention effective January 1, 2022 (The Joint Commission, 2023a). TJC mentioned that WPV recurrently goes unreported, indicating accurate rates of WPV are likely much higher than documented (The Joint Commission, 2021). All Joint Commission-accredited hospitals must employ updated and revised strategies that decrease instances of WPV (The Joint Commission, 2021). The Joint Commission (2021) stated that healthcare and social service workers were five times more likely to combat WPV than other workers, encompassing 73% of all nonfatal WPV events. Lim et al. (2022) revealed statistics showing that healthcare violence is progressively problematic regardless of where nurses work. Lim et al. also conferred that healthcare workers face a substantial challenge by being five times more likely than other occupations to sustain work-related injuries due to violence.

The data from this original qualitative study will help readers understand nurses' lived experiences with WPV and how these experiences extensively impacted the nurse's role. Bildik et al. (2022) mentioned that while WPV victimizes the individual, it affects the entire healthcare team and the quality of health services delivered. Ogboghodo and Okojie (2020) researched the prevalence and patterns of WPV among healthcare workers in Nigeria, with 83.7% of the 386 participants admitting to experiencing WPV, validating the need for a new perspective and proposed solutions to manage global WPV in healthcare effectively.

Significance of the Study

Nursing administration requires evidence in the form of data to show the negative impact that WPV has on nurses in healthcare institutions. Implementing programs that educate nurses on the proper handling of WPV, appropriate ways to report violence, and ways to obtain support after violence occurs are critical to the successful execution of zero-tolerance WPV policies. Additionally, by learning the perspective of the nurses who experience WPV, positive solutions can generate a cultural shift in the nursing profession, improving staff retention, and decreasing the cost of staff turnover.

The theoretical framework used for this study was Ida Jean Orlando's nursing process discipline theory (Orlando, 1961, as cited in Petiprin, 2023). Orlando's theory is founded on the concepts of the function of professional nursing, behaviors at patient presentation, immediate reaction, the nursing process discipline, and process improvement (Orlando, 1961, as cited in Petiprin, 2023). Based on what this researcher learned from Petiprin (2023), Orlando's theory applies to this study by discussing a nurse successfully navigating the care of patients susceptible to violence in distressing situations and how the nurse can meet their immediate needs. The results of this researcher's data contributed to nursing theory by ensuring nurse managers have adequately prepared nurses on the potential risks and various types of WPV in the healthcare setting and how to mitigate violence when it occurs. The outcomes generated by this researcher from this study's data may empower nurses to report incidents of WPV better and feel supported by nursing leadership with regulatory policies and procedures that foster a zero-tolerance policy for WPV.

Although research is ongoing to reduce WPV in healthcare, reliable solutions are needed to resolve this healthcare epidemic (Báez-León et al., 2016; Beattie et al., 2019; Bildik et al., 2022; Dadashzadeh et al., 2019; Doehring et al., 2023; Kiymaz & Koç, 2023; Lim et al., 2022; Moman et al., 2020; Nevels et al., 2020; Ogboghodo & Okojie, 2020). This researcher closed a gap in the existing literature regarding WPV solutions by detailing the nurses' experiences of WPV and strategies used to overcome them. The outcomes of Kiymaz & Koç's (2023) study supported the need for healthcare reform regarding violence against nurses to improve the healthcare environment and occupational commitment. This researcher offered meaningful potential solutions to the phenomenon of WPV after gaining the nurse's perspective on experiences with violence in healthcare.

Research Question

This researcher designed qualitative research using semi-structured interviews asking RNs open-ended questions exploring the research question: What are the lived experiences of nurses who have dealt with violence from patients, family members, and visitors? Polit and Beck (2021) defined *phenomenology* as a qualitative research approach in which the researcher aims to understand different ways people experience a phenomenon. This researcher investigated nurses' experiences with WPV to examine the phenomenon from a new perspective. To provide meaningful solutions to violence mitigation in healthcare, the individuals who experience it most deserve a crucial role in projected solutions.

Definition of Terms

This researcher incorporated the definition of terms section to maintain the reader's understanding of this researcher's approach to this qualitative study. Polit and Beck (2021) indicated that by describing vocabulary in qualitative research, the researcher attempts to make a qualitative study as rigorous, trustworthy, insightful, and valid as possible. This researcher limited confusion or misinterpretation of terms by clearly defining study terminology (Polit & Beck, 2021).

Occupational Safety and Health Administration (OSHA): Congress created the Occupational Safety and Health Act of 1970 to set and enforce standards that ensure safe and healthy working conditions and provide training, education, outreach, and assistance (Occupational Safety and Health Administration, n.d.).

***Qualitative research*:** Polit and Beck (2021) depicted qualitative research as an in-depth investigation of phenomena by collecting narrative materials using a research design.

***Registered nurse (RN)*:** The North Carolina Board of Nursing (2023) discussed that the nurse's role is to maintain health, prevent and manage illness, injury, and disability, and assist patients with dignity in dying. The North Carolina Board of Nursing clarified that the full scope of nursing is practiced by caring for clients in various settings, which is defined by the nursing process as assessing, planning, and implementing prescribed individualized and comprehensive treatments. According to the North Carolina Board of Nursing, registered nurses care for individuals, communities, and populations; they teach individuals how to care for themselves or family members who provide care at home. Nurses reassess interventions and treatments following medication administration, collaborating with the interdisciplinary team to holistically care for individuals as needed (North Carolina Board of Nursing, 2023).

***The Joint Commission (TJC)*:** assesses the safety of healthcare organizations, sets regulatory standards for quality of care and performance, and provides educational solutions for improving healthcare institutions globally (The Joint Commission, 2023b).

***Workplace violence (WPV)*:** Threats or acts of physical violence, verbal abuse, intimidation, hostility, harassment, and even homicide that occur while someone is at their place of employment (United States Department of Labor, n.d.).

Research Design

Polit and Beck (2021) indicated that qualitative research is a type of research that seeks to answer specific questions. Polit & Beck (2021, p. 45) described, "In qualitative studies, conceptual definitions of key phenomena may be a major end product, reflecting an intent to have the meaning of concepts defined by those being studied." Polit and Beck mentioned that qualitative research variables differ from quantitative research as they are not simply measured or defined. According to Polit and Beck, qualitative data is obtained by the researcher conversing with participants about the phenomenon, whereas quantitative data is numerical. This qualitative research focused on relationships between the phenomena of WPV and the nurses who experienced it (Polit & Beck, 2021). Guided by Polit and Beck, this researcher emphasized the experiences of WPV and searched for patterns and connections to illuminate the underlying meaning and dimensionality of WPV (Polit & Beck, 2021).

Polit and Beck (2021) described the need for qualitative research to compare and categorize relative patterns. This researcher selected participants of various ages with diverse nursing practice experiences to ensure that data accurately portrayed the nurses' experiences with WPV. Data analysis was guided by concept development through analysis of essential aspects noted in previous participant interviews (Dadashzadeh et al., 2019).

This researcher used a descriptive qualitative design method for this study. Through approximately 30-minute individually audio-recorded interviews, nurses described their experiences with WPV and how it affected them personally and professionally. This researcher used an emergent design for the study, with ongoing considerations based on the information learned from previous study participants (Polit & Beck, 2021). As this researcher gained insight into nurses' experiences with violence, various data collection strategies occurred, assisting the researcher in determining data saturation (Polit & Beck, 2021).

This researcher collected demographic data from all participants, including age, educational preparation, and work experience. A framework of predetermined interview questions guided participant discussions, and time was allotted for participants to elaborate on their experiences with WPV. This researcher asked the participants specific questions about their experiences with WPV, allowing the identification of trends in WPV occurrence. Guided by Polit and Beck (2021), this researcher studied the raw data and investigated the intuitive phenomenon of WPV against nurses in the healthcare setting.

Polit and Beck (2021) described the need for qualitative research to compare and categorize relative patterns. This researcher selected participants of various ages with diverse nursing backgrounds to ensure that data accurately portrayed nurses' experiences with WPV. Concept development guided data analysis by analyzing essential aspects noted in previous participant interviews (Dadashzadeh et al., 2019).

Assumptions and Limitations

Polit and Beck (2021) discussed that an assumption is a principle believed to be true without proof. Polit and Beck (2021, p. 8) described the constructivist paradigm as "taking apart old ideas... and putting ideas and structures together in new ways." Polit and Beck (2021, p. 8) also stated, "The constructivist paradigm assumes that knowledge is maximized when the distance between the researcher and those under study is minimized." Polit and Beck described qualitative research limitations as the subjectivity of information gathered and any variables that may limit the study's validity, credibility, or generalizability.

Assumptions

This researcher designed this research study on a constructive paradigm intended to increase our focus on the phenomenon of WPV (Polit & Beck, 2021). This researcher assumed that participants answered questions to the best of their ability, providing candid responses (Polit & Beck, 2021). This researcher assumed that the inclusion and exclusion criteria for the study sample were appropriate, ensuring all participants had experienced WPV from a licensed nurse's perspective in a healthcare setting. Additionally, this researcher assumed no ethical constraints or circumstances would persuade biased study participation (Polit & Beck, 2021).

This researcher kept all interviews objective by keeping an audio-recorded reflective journal of personal beliefs or biases that could threaten the validity of responses (Polit & Beck, 2021). This researcher assumed that many professions might find the generalizability of study findings applicable and helpful (Polit & Beck, 2021). Although the goal of this study was not comparative, this researcher had planned for the possibility of comparisons by choosing diverse study participants who met the study's inclusion and exclusion criteria (Polit & Beck, 2021).

Limitations

Although this researcher yielded rich information showing a specific dimension of WPV experiences, limitations were out of this researcher's control (Polit & Beck, 2021). The first limitation included the researcher conducting a small-scale study in a remote location. Due to the study's sensitivity, participants may have felt biased in answering questions about how WPV was handled at their workplaces. Another study limitation was the participant's inability to recollect the exact circumstances surrounding certain WPV events. This researcher continued to collect data until data saturation was achieved; however, a small sample size may have been an additional study limitation.

Organization of the Remainder of the Study

In Chapter 1, this researcher reviewed the background, need, purpose, and significance of this qualitative master's research study that explored the lived experiences of nurses who encountered WPV and how it impacted their role as a nurse. This researcher used a semi-structured, open-ended interview approach to address the research question: What are nurses' experiences with WPV? This researcher provided definitions of critical terms and explained the study's research design (Polit & Beck, 2021).

In Chapter 2, this researcher will provide an in-depth review of the current literature regarding WPV and how this affected the nurse's role. In Chapter 3, this researcher will discuss the basic qualitative methodology used in this research. In Chapter 4, this researcher will explain the analysis of data collected from study participants and themes and codes established in participant interviews. In Chapter 5, this researcher will examine how research findings will improve and mitigate WPV against nurses in the acute care setting by implementing successful strategies learned by nurses.

CHAPTER 2. LITERATURE REVIEW

WPV has been a topic of discussion for global healthcare leaders for many years, as supported by extensive literature and many studies that examine different aspects of this topic and search for ways to mitigate and end violence (Báez-León et al., 2016; Beattie et al., 2019; Bildik et al., 2022; Dadashzadeh et al., 2019; Doehring et al., 2023; Kiymaz & Koç, 2023; Lim et al., 2022; Moman et al., 2020; Nevels et al., 2020; Ogboghodo & Okojie, 2020). This researcher examined how WPV affects the nurses' personal and professional lives, job satisfaction, retention, and the level of support they experience as victims of WPV.

Methods of Searching

Research for the supporting literature occurred through the University of Mount Olive's (UMO) online research platform provided by Moye Library. The Cumulative Index and Nursing Allied Health Literature (CINALH) research database yielded valuable supporting literature. This researcher limited database searches to nursing, medicine, and allied health disciplines. Furthermore, this researcher narrowed the literature search by limiting the publication dates between 2016 and 2023. This researcher used keywords such as *workplace violence*, *violence against nurses from patients*, *violence against nurses from family members*, *safety against violence in healthcare*, and *global workplace violence in healthcare*. This researcher confined the search to include only scholarly, peer-reviewed, full-text articles in English.

Theoretical Orientation for the Study

The theoretical orientation used for this study was the descriptive phenomenological research developed by Husserl and Heidegger (Polit & Beck, 2021).

Using phenomenological analysis, this researcher was primarily interested in depicting the nurses' experiences with WPV (Polit & Beck, 2021). This researcher chose this approach to consider what each study participant remembered, felt, saw, heard, believed, and experienced through semi-structured interviews (Polit & Beck, 2021).

Review of the Literature

Dafny and Beccaria (2020) discussed how nurses frequently perceive violence in healthcare as a routine part of their job. This researcher designed a study to explore how WPV affects nurses, and this researcher used the literature review to fuse data from the chosen articles to expose themes identified with WPV (Polit & Beck, 2021). Polit and Beck aided this researcher's literature review to facilitate the reader's understanding and evaluation of evidence supporting the current knowledge about WPV.

WPV: A Healthcare Epidemic

Báez-León et al. (2016) emphasized addressing WPV in healthcare after The Joint Commission (TJC) released a Sentinel Event Alert, reporting that approximately 75% of workplace assaults occur annually in healthcare and social services settings alone. Báez-León et al. revealed that components that likely contributed to violence included patients with altered mental status, mental illness, cognitive decline, delirium, intoxication, and individuals in stressful situations with poor prognoses. Báez-León et al. specified that TJC set standards for leadership, individuals, and environmental factors to safeguard persons of an organization against WPV.

Báez-León et al. (2016) indicated that employees should review incident logs and WPV policies to understand likely risk factors for violence and address the most common occurrences of WPV. Báez-León et al. identified the need for healthcare facilities to conduct drills for all employees to learn what to do during an active shooter emergency. Báez-León et al. detailed that policy and procedure should specifically discuss the code of conduct, and nurses should recognize when violence escalates.

Although total avoidance of violence in the healthcare setting is impossible, Báez-León et al. (2016) suggested using a three-pronged approach that addresses prevention, reporting, and reaction to minimize the impacts of violence on staff. Other safeguards include self-locking doors, metal detectors, not allowing visitors to enter the facility on a 24-hour basis, security cameras, security staff, and encouraging staff to report instances of WPV (Báez-León et al., 2016). Báez-León et al. declared that any occurrence of WPV offers an opportunity to analyze system failures and help prevent further violence in the future. According to Báez-León et al., there is a critical need for adequate funding to support the safety of staff and patients. WPV tarnishes a facility's reputation and has lasting trauma on those who suffer from violence.

Global Concerns for WPV

Ogboghodo and Okojie (2020) assessed the frequency and patterns of WPV among healthcare workers in Tertiary Health facilities in Benin City, Nigeria, the capital of Edo State. Ogboghodo and Okojie used a descriptive, cross-sectional study design to assess the prevalence and patterns of WPV in healthcare. Ogboghodo and Okojie conducted the study to propose suggestions to improve staff safety and enhance patient care. Ogboghodo and Okojie selected study participants using the stratified sampling technique, and Ogboghodo and Okojie distributed a confidential, structured questionnaire to assess incidences and types of WPV. According to Ogboghodo and Okojie, of the 386 participants, 285 individuals (83.7%) admitted to suffering from WPV, 73.8% experienced physical violence, 69.2% experienced verbal violence, 34.5% experienced sexual violence, 34.5% endured emotional violence in the workplace. In the studied group, Ogboghodo and Okojie demonstrated physical violence as the most prevalent form of WPV. Ogboghodo and Okojie's research validated the need to gain a new perspective on WPV and regulate WPV interventions globally in the healthcare setting.

Nurses Combat Pre-Hospital WPV in Iran

Dadashzadeh et al. (2019) discussed that little research is available to address the experiences of pre-hospital nurses with WPV in Iran. Dadashzadeh et al. used semi-structured interviews to collect data for a descriptive qualitative study involving 19 male nurses working in a pre-hospital setting in Iran. According to Dadashzadeh et al., nurses are now among pre-hospital providers due to insufficient emergency medical technicians (EMTs) in Iran. However, they do not receive any specialized training for this type of work in nursing school. Dadashzadeh et al. mentioned that identifying how these pre-hospital nurses dealt with WPV helped develop guidelines to reduce WPV in this setting.

Dadashzadeh et al. (2019) chose a descriptive qualitative study design to explore the phenomenon of WPV in Iranian pre-hospital nurses. Dadashzadeh et al. conducted the study between December 2017 and September 2018 in East Azerbaijan Province, Iran, which covers approximately 45 square kilometers. Dadashzadeh et al.

explained that there are 41 urban and 61 interurban ambulance stations and one air emergency station with 450 personnel who provide pre-hospital care in this area. Dadashzadeh et al. mentioned that only men could work in the pre-hospital setting due to Iran's unique culturally-based rules and policies.

Dadashzadeh et al. (2019) applied study eligibility criteria that yielded 19 male nurses who held a baccalaureate or master's degree in nursing, had at least two years of pre-hospital work experience, and willingness to participate in the research. Dadashzadeh et al. used a purposive sampling method, and the initial participant had extensive pre-hospital expertise to aid the researchers in narrowing questions to focus on the main themes or clear any ambiguity from other participants. Dadashzadeh et al. conducted interviews privately, obtaining demographic information, and then inquired about the occurrences of WPV and the outcomes. Dadashzadeh et al. completed twenty-four interviews with a mean interview duration of 65 minutes (35 to 120 minutes), with secondary interviews taking a mean of 28 minutes (15 to 39 minutes). Dadashzadeh et al. transcribed participant interviews, reviewed interviews multiple times, and labeled the interviews with themes until no new data emerged.

Dadashzadeh et al. (2019) utilized manual methods for data analysis. The mean age of participants was 36 years (28-46), with an average work experience of 12 years (3-20), according to Dadashzadeh et al., 2019. Dadashzadeh et al. discussed the four themes that emerged as strategies for handling WPV. Dadashzadeh et al. identified these themes as no reaction to WPV (tolerance and acceptance), situational management (patient and scene management), confrontation (direct and indirect), and escaping the scene.

Dadashzadeh et al. (2019) revealed that some nurses tolerated WPV due to fear of escalating violence, fear of harm from WPV, fear of delays in reaching the scene of an incident, working in isolated locations, and fear of legal issues from perpetrators of violence. Dadashzadeh et al. confirmed that participants admitted they were more tolerant of verbal and psychological violence than physical violence. Nurses with more work experience stated that this strategy of tolerating simple verbal or psychological violence prevented violence from becoming out of control or dangerous to the staff or patients (Dadashzadeh et al., 2019).

Dadashzadeh et al. (2019) documented that several nurses reported that they expected acts of violence from patients, family members, and bystanders. They responded by promptly tending to their patients to diffuse violent situations, according to Dadashzadeh et al., 2019. Nurses reported that this method frequently reduced tension but was ineffective for intense acts of violence (Dadashzadeh et al., 2019). Dadashzadeh et al. also said that nurses expressed that promoting scene safety, reducing bystander stress, and focusing on the scene's elements were helpful strategies for managing WPV. Dadashzadeh et al. recognized that nurses occasionally used confrontation of WPV by nurses, more commonly, less experienced staff, primarily due to high fatigue, stress, and severity of violence. Dadashzadeh et al. mentioned indirect methods of confronting violence were having influential elders present on the scene or police force to de-escalate violence from bystanders.

Dadashzadeh et al. (2019) disclosed that some nurses admitted occasionally reacting to violence, becoming mutually violent in return; however, most discussed using self-defense methods, tackling an attacker, or mutual combat. Dadashzadeh et al. reported that when the pre-hospital nurses sensed extreme danger or potential for severe violence, they exercised extreme caution when entering a scene and continuously considered escape strategies. Dadashzadeh et al. believed that participants noted disadvantages to this strategy, such as escaping the scene without the patient.

Dadashzadeh et al. (2019) recounted that tolerating violence in hopes that it would not escalate had negative psychological impacts on the staff. This increased job dissatisfaction, and many nurses left their professions (Dadashzadeh et al., 2019). Dadashzadeh et al. conferred that situational management of WPV was the most commonly used method of dealing with WPV, which often reduced tension at the scene but simultaneously left less time to render aid to the patient. Dadashzadeh et al. acknowledged that confrontation of violence by nurses themselves increased personal injuries among staff. However, Dadashzadeh et al. described indirect methods, such as having police intervention, as challenging because frequently, police were not present at the onset of violence. Unfortunately, due to violence, Dadashzadeh et al. explained that personnel had occasions when they had to leave the scene and abandon the patient, increasing rates of morbidity and mortality.

Dadashzadeh et al. (2019) acknowledged a lack of guidelines for mitigating WPV in Iranian pre-hospital settings and explained that the responsibility is that of the Iranian Ministry of Health. Dadashzadeh et al. mentioned that challenges in the pre-hospital setting require education and strategies to better prepare nurses for these scenarios. Dadashzadeh et al. discussed simultaneously dispatching pre-hospital staff and police to scenes where violence can be expected, such as a crime scene.

Dadashzadeh et al. described the importance of safeguarding nurses from WPV in all healthcare settings and ensuring patients are offered the best chance of survival and recovery.

Violence Across Healthcare Disciplines

Managing pain is a fundamental patient right and a crucial priority for nurses providing patient-centered care. Moman et al. (2020) explained that as healthcare teams learn to navigate providing adequate pain control through an opioid crisis, many efforts may go unnoticed by patients, causing an escalation of patient violence if methods of pain control are not to the patient's satisfaction. Moman et al. studied the prevalence and characteristics of WPV among pain-management providers, including physicians, residents, fellows, nurse practitioners, physician assistants, and psychologists, at the 2019 American Academy of Pain Medicine annual meeting in Denver, Colorado. Additional objectives included how individuals perpetrated violence and threats and the association of high-risk factors associated with WPV (Moman et al., 2020). Moman et al. administered written survey questionnaires to all 70 attendees and asked them to complete them during a one-hour educational session, with 58 participants submitting responses.

Moman et al. (2020) reported that results yielded the mean age of providers as 47.5 years, with 23 (41.1%) of the providers who replied being female. Moman et al. described that of the survey participants, 82.8% said they had called the police at least once within the last year due to a disruptive patient, and 68.4 % recounted threats of bodily harm. Moman et al. stated that five participants reported being physically assaulted, with 68.4% saying they are threatened at least once annually with violence. Moman et al. noted that providers conveyed that most threats are due to worker's compensation claims, disability requests, and automobile accidents. Moman et al. considered factors cited by perpetrators of violence, including dissatisfaction with care, chronic pain, intoxication, declining mental health conditions, and characteristics of the providers. Moman et al. discovered that poor violence prevention protocols are associated with higher rates of violence and that urban areas are 1.5 times more likely to experience indirect physical violence.

Moman et al. (2020) mentioned limitations such as utilizing self-reporting of WPV. A cross-sectional survey might identify causes of violence but not determine the contributory constituents of violence. Additionally, Moman et al. described that this research was generalized to some clinical sites where patients with chronic pain obtain care. Moman et al. indicated that it is crucial to identify high-risk clinical scenarios, and the need for further research to reduce WPV is ongoing.

Negative Effects of WPV

Lim et al. (2022) stated that WPV has become a worldwide concern and threatens society's well-being. They also indicated that WPV in healthcare continues to increase with rising workloads, excessive stress, and increased social and economic uncertainties. Lim et al. identified risk factors and the implications of WPV in the healthcare setting and highlighted the need for collaborative forces that prevent and mitigate WPV.

Lim et al. (2022) presented a meta-analysis of 47 observational studies demonstrating that 62.4% of healthcare workers experienced some form of WPV. Lim et al. mentioned that verbal abuse was the most common method of WPV (61.2%), followed by psychological violence (50.8%), threats (39.5%), physical violence (13.7%), and sexual harassment (6.3%). Lim et al. identified more recent WPV instances, including cyberbullying, humiliation, defamation, and unlawful video recording in a healthcare setting. Lim et al. emphasized risk factors perpetuating violence in the healthcare setting, including environmental factors like overcrowding, long wait times, and cultural and language differences. According to Lim et al., the attitudes and behaviors of patients, family members, and visitors under immeasurable emotional stress may perhaps also cause WPV.

Lim et al. (2022) reported that individuals who experience violence are more prone to experience post-traumatic stress disorder (PTSD), depression, irritability, sleep disorders, and difficulty concentrating. Lim et al. clarified that many healthcare workers are choosing to leave their respective fields due to violence because perpetrators of violence have no action taken against them. Individuals may be singled out as victims of violence or retaliation if they choose to file reports. Lim et al. reviewed an extensive need to expand WPV prevention strategies to reduce the adverse psychological effects on healthcare workers. Lim et al. observed that individual healthcare settings need specific comprehensive WPV guidelines personalized to their department needs supported by evidence-based research and national organizational guidelines.

Lim et al. (2022) cited that it is imperative to advocate for WPV awareness, incorporate zero-tolerance policies, improve WPV educational programs, integrate WPV prevention measures in the accreditation process, and offer support to victims of WPV. Lim et al. explained a need for collaborative efforts such as financial support from the community, non-governmental organizations (NGOs), and business corporations to collaboratively and comprehensively address WPV in healthcare. Lim et al. declared that WPV is confronted best by creating a united front that includes the government's policies, healthcare management, healthcare workers, professional organizations, NGOs, and the community.

Violence Affects Retention

Kiymaz and Koç (2023) reviewed a variety of violence ED nurses are routinely subjected to and how it affected them physically, psychologically, and socially, causing them to consider resignation. Kiymaz and Koç noted causative factors that nurses cannot control, such as overcrowding, long wait times, understaffing, and workloads in the ED that place them at higher risk of being victimized by WPV. A sample size of 169 ED nurses with at least one year of experience participated in a questionnaire about the violence they were exposed to, occupational commitment, and their intention to resign (Kiymaz & Koç, 2023). Kiymaz and Koç determined that as nurses' exposure to violence increased, their occupational commitment decreased, increasing their intent to resign.

Perceptions of Safety

Bildik et al. (2022) assessed the connection between working conditions, safety, confidence perception, and sociodemographic characteristics of physicians working in assorted EDs in Turkey from January 2021 through January 2022. Bildik et al. used a two-part online survey to inquire about participant demographics, characteristics, working conditions, the type of facility where they practiced, how safe they felt, and how confident they felt when faced with violence. Bildik et al.

applied a 10-point Turkish scale with proven validity and reliability to gather information about safety and confidence.

Bildik et al. (2022) surveyed 405 participants and received 402 responses. The median age of providers was 29 (26-36) years, with 211 males and 191 females (Bildik et al., 2022). Bildik et al. observed that general practitioners comprised 49% of respondents, 76.6% of physicians reported working in the city center, and an average of six physicians (3-10) worked each shift. Bildik et al. described that the average number of patients seen daily in these EDs ranged between 500 and 1,000. Bildik et al. noted that among participants, 42.5% of providers had 1-5 years of work experience. The median age of participants with less than one year of experience was 39, according to Bildik et al., 2022.

Bildik et al. (2022) stated that 307 (76.4%) participants reported experiencing verbal violence, 61(15.2%) participants said they had suffered both physical and verbal violence, and 30 (7.5%) participants stated they had not experienced any form of WPV. In this study, "physicians with less than one year of work experience had significantly lower Safety and Confidence Scale for Health Professionals (SCSHP) scores than those with more than one year of work experience" (Bildik et al., 2022, p. 12). According to Bildik et al., general practitioners also had lower SCSHP scores than specialists; male or married physicians had higher SCSHP scores than female or unmarried physicians. Bildik et al. noticed that environmental factors, such as the number of patients seen daily, geographical region, urban versus rural facility location, and the presence of security personnel, did not affect the provider's feelings of safety and confidence. Consistent with Bildik et al., physicians in the ED who have less work experience, are unmarried, and females feel less safe and less confident about encountering and handling WPV. Bildik et al. conferred that administrative and educational interventions should support employees in improving their perception of safety and confidence when facing WPV.

Policy Against Violence

Doehring et al. (2023) completed a five-month survey in an urban ED serving approximately 100,000 patients annually, yielding that WPV is common, occurring almost daily, and frequently involves racist, sexist, or homophobic bias. Doehring et al. data revealed that men are often the perpetrators of violence, with most victims being nurses. With daily occurrences of violence, and 20% of these instances involving physical violence, the rates of safety incidents are alarming, according to Doehring et al. Doehring et al. stated that healthcare needs policy change at the local, state, and national levels to reduce staggering rates of WPV.

Relationships Between Trauma and Violence

Beattie et al. (2019) considered multi-factorial obstacles when encountering WPV in healthcare and numerous ways to conquer them. Beattie et al. examined WPV perpetrated by clients in healthcare towards nurses, reported the conclusions of a study on WPV from individuals who had experienced adverse childhood events (ACEs), incorporated neurophysiology advances in understanding violence, and discussed a trauma-informed approach to providing patient care. Beattie et al. distinguished risk factors that staff believed perpetuated acts of aggressive behavior, which included poor environmental settings, long ED wait times, overcrowding, excessive noise, lack of privacy and space, inadequate staffing, poor patient-staff communication, firm visitation policies, noticeable favoritism, and perceived or fundamental staff incompetence.

The ACE Study enriched the understanding of the relationships between ACEs and their influence on the individual's welfare as an adult (Felitti et al., 1988, as cited in Beattie et al., 2019). Beattie et al. (2019) noted that by studying ACEs such as psychological, physical, and sexual abuse, exposure to violence, exposure to substance abuse, exposure to mental illness, and having family members incarcerated, nurses had an increased capacity to recognize possible offenders of WPV. Over half of the ACE study participants reported having >/= 1 of these ACEs, while 6.2% disclosed >/= 4 exposures (Felitti et al., 1988, cited in Beattie et al., 2019). "Exposure to ACEs affects brain development and leads to a cascade of biological changes and stress responses which are highly associated with mental health conditions including unresolved anger, post-traumatic stress disorder (PTSD), and substance use disorders" (Forkey et al., 2014 as cited in Beattie et al., 2019, p. 118). Beattie et al. expressed that hyperarousal frequently appears as a method of self-preservation immediately following trauma; however, this coping mechanism used over a lifetime may interfere with the individual's ability to assess potential threats or feelings that jeopardize safety appropriately.

Beattie et al. (2019) reported that safety is often viewed differently among individuals; however, the body's response to threats of safety activates the sympathetic nervous system (SNS), or fight or flight defense mechanism, in response to threats or perceived threats to one's safety. In contrast, the parasympathetic nervous system (PNS) regulates bodily functions involved in social exchanges and communication “such as facial expression, vocalization, hearing, listening, and breathing” (Beattie et al., 2019, p. 119). The dorsal vagal pathway regulates the internal organs below the diaphragm and is adept at triggering the body’s immobilization defense response (“dissociation, freeze, and fold”) (Beattie et al., 2019, p. 119). If a “perceived or real threat is detected, such as physical/emotional stress, trauma, illness or unfamiliar environment, the SNS is ‘recruited’ to fight or flee” (Beattie et al., 2019, p. 119). Beattie et al. described that this is why social interactions from healthcare workers must be perceived as safe and pleasant engagements, decreasing the likelihood of perceived threats to safety that cause the behaviors of individuals to escalate.

Beattie et al. (2019) used an explanatory study as part of a more extensive descriptive study examining staff’s experiences of WPV and the guidance used to manage it. Beattie et al. conducted this research in Australia, with 136 hospitals being approached, including facility and participant diversity. Beattie et al. used experienced staff in high-risk areas to conduct participant interviews, and these staff members dictated interviews verbatim to allow researchers an extensive review. Beattie et al. employed an electronic data management system, allowing the researchers to identify themes among the occurrences of WPV. Ninety-nine volunteers participated in the interview process, conducting 33 individual interviews and performing 21 group interviews (Beattie et al., 2019). Beattie et al. noted that among the participants, 69.7% were female and 30.3% male, with interviews lasting an average of 28.5 minutes. The participants in Beattie et al. were mainly employed at administrative levels, working in regional hospitals (57.6%), city hospitals (39.4%), and specialist hospitals (3%).

Beattie et al. (2019) noted that verbal aggression was a common form of WPV identified among participants, with healthcare workers acknowledging high-stress situations likely precipitating verbal acts of violence from patients, families, and visitors. Beattie et al. emphasized that participants felt that ACEs and previous traumas, such as being ill-treated while previously institutionalized, may have caused increased agitation toward staff. Additionally, Beattie et al. described that staff providing firm instructions, patients experiencing feelings of confinement, and waking up from anesthetic medications also led patients to increased distress and the likelihood of hostility.

Beattie et al. (2019) described trauma-informed care as an endorsed model for hospitals to boost a mentally healthy workplace for patients and employees concurrently. Beattie et al. discussed that by incorporating trauma assessments into patient care, the nurse could further understand individual patients and their specific trauma-related triggers frequently preceding escalating behaviors. Beattie et al. recommended calmly engaging with patients at the first signs of agitation, including them in patient-centered care, and providing adequate information, medication, treatments, and appropriate follow-up to decrease the likelihood of WPV. According to Beattie et al., staff participation in resilience training, notifying patients of unforeseen treatment delays, reacting appropriately when escalation occurs, and boundary setting improved positive patient-staff communication.

Beattie et al. (2019) indicated that nurses recognized that patients and family members were often tense upon arrival to the healthcare setting. Beattie et al. discussed how stress prompts the body's SNS activation, which slows down the individual's ability to regulate their thought process, emotions, and behaviors. Beattie et al. described that the SNS activation process unconsciously places these individuals at higher risk of initiating aggression and violence. Beattie et al. described helpful sensory-based interventions such as guided imagery, weighted blankets, decreased lighting, and providing lotion or oil, which may enhance patient engagement. Beattie et al. explained that decreasing emotional reactivity and increasing social engagement are crucial to reducing WPV. Furthermore, Beattie et al. mentioned that the nurse's tone of voice, body language, active listening, facial expressions, and posture should demonstrate an open and trusting demeanor with patients and their loved ones. According to Beattie et al., emphasizing empathy and individualized care helps meet needs and not re-traumatize hospitalized patients.

Beattie et al. (2019) described WPV as a multi-faceted problem, and research participants suggested implementing a trauma-informed recovery model program to help prevent and manage WPV in their healthcare settings. Beattie et al. stated that using a trauma-informed approach to patient care makes staff more aware of specific ACEs, which may improve communication and decrease the likelihood of patient violence. Beattie et al. conveyed that although WPV remains a critical healthcare problem, understanding and applying current neuroscience and implementing a cultural shift of trauma-informed care reduces instances of WPV.

Mitigation Until Legislation

Nevels et al. (2020) acknowledged that healthcare workers are at higher risk of experiencing WPV and often perceive violence as a routine part of their duties. Nevels et al. expressed that, unfortunately, these feelings of complacency often lead to an underreporting of WPV occurrences. Nevels et al. recommended using a buddy system in high-risk situations to aid in providing patient care to combative patients and reducing the likelihood of WPV.

Nevels et al. (2020) exclaimed that employers have a moral obligation to keep staff safe and manage cost control related to instances of WPV. Nevels et al. conveyed that workers' compensation claims are motivational factors for reducing WPV; however, these claims costs are minimal compared to the overall cost of injuries and fatalities that WPV can cause. Nevels et al. implied that addressing gaps in WPV prevention and management strategies is worthy of financial investment and collaboration from labor groups, unions, insurance companies, and governmental agencies.

Nevels et al. (2020, p. 42) revealed, “Risk reduction using engineering controls is the most widely used method when addressing WPV.” These strategies include “parameter security with fencing, walls, outdoor locking egress doorways and metal detectors, which have all proven successful for restricting entry” (Nevels et al., 2020, p. 42). Succeeding the interior of the facility should include “closed-circuit television in conjunction with security staff, employee panic buttons, and illumination improvements to provide better workplace oversight and emergency communication” (Nevels et al., 2020, p. 42). Nevels et al. revealed that paramount skills for staff, such as situational awareness, de-escalation techniques, and recognition of an unraveling situation, are all critical components in WPV prevention. Nevels et al. discussed that prevention-by-observation requires staff to utilize situational awareness to prevent the probability of violence with the hopes of controlling radical behaviors before an individual escalates and becomes out of control. Nevels et al. mentioned that identifying previous offenders of violence is an added strategy for protecting staff and promoting the facility's overall safety.

Nevels et al. (2020, p. 43) emphasized, "One weakness of healthcare violence prevention programs lies in the balance between patient satisfaction and employee protection." Nevels et al. mentioned that hospitals must obtain acceptable scores on Hospital Consumer Assessment of Healthcare Providers and Systems (HCAHPS) surveys to receive federal funding. Although the HCAHPS ensures transparency and accountability of healthcare institutions, many healthcare workers have described them as counterproductive in reducing occasions of WPV (Nevels et al., 2020). Nevels et al. expressed that nurses are responsible for providing quality patient care and excellent customer service, which may decrease their proficiency with WPV control measures and reporting criteria.

Nevels et al. (2020) declared that employee safety is essential for management to recognize and accentuate by leadership as just as vital as patient safety. "Training efforts by the employer and proper goal-setting strategies by management are necessary to keep the message consistent and clear, and delivered with the support of the caregivers in mind" (Nevels et al., 2020, p. 43). "If the organizational culture is built around safe work practices and solid management leadership, integration of an effective WPV prevention program should garner the support of its stakeholders and protect the safety and health of the healthcare professional" (Nevels et al., 2020, p. 43).

Nevels et al. (2020) voiced that WPV has captured the attention of diverse labor groups, healthcare organizations, and accreditation bodies, pursuing the issue of violence and providing support to pass legislative requirements that require organizations to keep healthcare workers safe. Nevels et al. described that due to the lengthy nature of the legislative process, the principles of risk assessment, the establishment of multiple layers of WPV control, and employees' heightened awareness of WPV would all be critical strategies in WPV reduction. According to Nevels et al., litigation will likely continue to result from ongoing occurrences of WPV where employees are injured or killed. Pending a standard practice implementation against WPV, Nevels et al. explained multiple valuable methods to aid healthcare workers in strategies to reduce and mitigate occurrences of WPV.

Synthesis of the Research Findings

The authors included in this literature review highlighted the occupational safety concerns of nurses with such frequent occurrences of WPV (Báez-León et al., 2016; Beattie et al., 2019; Bildik et al., 2022; Dadashzadeh et al., 2019; Doehring et al., 2023; Kiymaz & Koç, 2023; Lim et al., 2022; Moman et al., 2020; Nevels et al., 2020; Ogboghodo & Okojie, 2020). One stance mentioned by researchers was policy reform surrounding WPV and how decreasing WPV increases nurses' occupational commitment to their profession (Doehring et al., 2023; Kiymaz & Koç, 2023; Ogboghodo & Okojie, 2020). Other concerns regarding nurses' commitment to their profession tie into patient safety and patient outcomes: If experienced nurses continue to leave acute care roles, how does this negatively impact the quality of care (Báez-León et al., 2016; Beattie et al., 2019; Bildik et al., 2022; Dadashzadeh et al., 2019; Doehring et al., 2023; Kiymaz & Koç, 2023; Lim et al., 2022; Moman et al., 2020; Nevels et al., 2020; Ogboghodo & Okojie, 2020)?

Solutions are implemented to mitigate instances of WPV, yet few have yielded successful results (Báez-León et al., 2016; Beattie et al., 2019; Bildik et al., 2022; Dadashzadeh et al., 2019; Doehring et al., 2023; Kiymaz & Koç, 2023; Lim et al., 2022; Moman et al., 2020; Nevels et al., 2020; Ogboghodo & Okojie, 2020). Lim et al. (2022) declared that a collaborative effort from management and colleagues is needed to support nurses dealing with WPV in healthcare effectively. Individual areas require specific guidelines from evidence-based research to establish practical, acceptable, and sustainable violence prevention plans (Báez-León et al., 2016; Beattie et al., 2019; Bildik et al., 2022; Dadashzadeh et al., 2019; Doehring et al., 2023; Kiymaz & Koç, 2023; Lim et al., 2022; Moman et al., 2020; Nevels et al., 2020; Ogboghodo & Okojie, 2020). Lim et al. indicated that supporting international and regional professional organizations, councils, and associations is essential to decreasing WPV, advocating for WPV awareness, and implementing accreditation procedures that prevent WPV.

Critique of Previous Research Methods

Each research study has strengths, limitations, and proposals for ongoing research. The researchers of qualitative studies used descriptive, cross-sectional, and observational approaches to gather data (Doehring et al., 2023; Lim et al., 2022;

Moman et al., 2020; Ogboghodo & Okojie, 2020). Kiymaz and Koç (2023) used a multi-method, collecting quantitative research data using scales and surveys developed to assess nurses' intention to resign or remain at their current jobs and qualitative methods to determine how nurses felt about exposure to WPV.

The strengths of the supporting literature include the recognition that WPV is a global problem for nurses across all healthcare disciplines requiring policy reform (Báez-León et al., 2016; Beattie et al., 2019; Bildik et al., 2022; Dadashzadeh et al., 2019; Doehring et al., 2023; Kiymaz & Koç, 2023; Lim et al., 2022; Moman et al., 2020; Nevels et al., 2020; Ogboghodo & Okojie, 2020). Limitations mentioned in the literature review included collaborative efforts and responsibility sharing from all levels, necessary financial support, management's dedication to WPV prevention, nurses' commitment to updating awareness and knowledge of WPV, and the inability to generalize WPV policies (Báez-León et al., 2016; Beattie et al., 2019; Bildik et al., 2022; Dadashzadeh et al., 2019; Doehring et al., 2023; Kiymaz & Koç, 2023; Lim et al., 2022; Moman et al., 2020; Nevels et al., 2020; Ogboghodo & Okojie, 2020).

Summary

The review of available current literature warrants the ongoing concern regarding nurses' experiences with WPV (Báez-León et al., 2016; Beattie et al., 2019; Bildik et al., 2022; Dadashzadeh et al., 2019; Doehring et al., 2023; Kiymaz & Koç, 2023; Lim et al., 2022; Moman et al., 2020; Nevels et al., 2020; Ogboghodo & Okojie, 2020). The researchers of the current literature highlighted likely reasons for WPV affecting nurses' satisfaction, commitment to occupation, and intention to resign (Kiymaz & Koç, 2023; Lim et al., 2022). Researchers also emphasized the need for additional awareness concerning WPV, strategies nurses can use to de-escalate violent situations, and the need for policy reform to improve WPV in the healthcare setting globally (Báez-León et al., 2016; Beattie et al., 2019; Bildik et al., 2022; Dadashzadeh et al., 2018; Doehring et al., 2023; Kiymaz & Koç, 2023; Lim et al., 2022; Moman et al., 2020; Nevels et al., 2020; Ogboghodo & Okojie, 2020).

In Chapter 3, this researcher will offer a thorough review of the qualitative study design used to explore the lived experiences of acute care nurses and their lived experiences with WPV. This researcher aimed to generate knowledge about WPV that can be useful in assorted settings (Polit & Beck, 2021). This researcher will also discuss reflexivity, which safeguards against personal bias in study results (Polit & Beck, 2021).

CHAPTER 3. METHODOLOGY

In this chapter, this researcher will discuss the study's purpose, the research question, and the step-by-step methods and procedures used to enable future researchers to replicate the study. This researcher describes the phenomenological study approach in detail in this section (Polit & Beck, 2021). This researcher utilized sampling for this research study to find a typical representation of WPV experiences among nurses and possibly form associations among different dimensions of nursing practice (Polit & Beck, 2021). This researcher will describe the study's methods, including participant selection and data collection, and explain how this researcher analyzed data in the procedures section (Polit & Beck, 2021). In this chapter, this researcher will also review the semi-structured, open-ended interviews conducted with study participants. While conducting this research study, this researcher considered ethical concerns, which will also be described in this chapter (Polit & Beck, 2021).

Purpose of the Study

The researcher designed this qualitative phenomenological study to explore nurses' experiences with WPV in a healthcare setting from the nurse's perspective. Understanding how WPV influences nurses as individuals and professionals could significantly improve healthcare workers' safety globally. This research is critical to the nursing field as it involves staff and patient safety, affects the quality of patient care, and could improve nursing staff fulfillment and retention. Additionally, this research could assist nursing management in planning educational curriculums to restructure violence mitigation and implement a zero-tolerance policy for WPV in healthcare.

Research Question

This researcher designed this qualitative study to use Husserl and Heidegger's approach to phenomenology (as cited by Polit & Beck, 2021). This researcher used semi-structured, open-ended interview questions to explore the research question: What are the lived experiences of nurses who have dealt with workplace violence from patients, family members, and visitors? This researcher aimed to propose new solutions for WPV by investigating the issue from a unique perspective.

Research Design

The researcher designed this basic qualitative study to use a descriptive phenomenology method (Polit & Beck, 2021, p. 478), supported by the theoretical framework of Ida Jean Orlando's nursing process discipline theory (Orlando, 1961, as cited in Petiprin, 2023). This researcher chose a descriptive phenomenological approach to emphasize portrayals of human experiences and describe what we know as humans (Polit & Beck, 2021). "Descriptive phenomenologists insist on the careful description of ordinary conscious experience of everyday life" (Polit & Beck, 2021, p. 478). Conducting approximately 30-minute audio-recorded, semi-structured interviews allowed themes to emerge with nurses who experience WPV from patients, family members, and visitors.

This researcher chose to examine how WPV impacts nurses as individuals and professionals and to see if they felt adequate support from leadership at their respective institutions. Throughout the interviews, this researcher bracketed or identified and held any possible preconceived notions in an audio-recorded reflexive journal with clarification on personal feelings or biases (Polit & Beck, 2021). This researcher performed bracketing to separate the researcher's emotions from the data analysis.

This research study is supported by the nursing process discipline theory by Ida Jean Orlando because it explains that the nurse's role is to meet the patient's immediate need for help (Orlando, 1961, as cited in Petiprin, 2023). This researcher learned that Orlando's theory specifically stated that patient behaviors might not be congruent with their need, and behaviors may be inappropriate, often used as a cry for help (Orlando, 1961, as cited in Petiprin, 2023). Using Orlando's theory, the nurse can assess the immediate behavior, reactions that require nursing intervention, and ways to improve the behavior (Orlando, 1961, as cited in Petiprin, 2023). Using Orlando's theory, the nurse has responded to an individual suffering, experiences feelings of hopelessness, and can avoid, diminish, or alleviate those feelings with nursing interventions (Orlando, 1961, as cited in Petiprin, 2023).

The data collected from the semi-structured interviews yielded critical information that answered the research question about nurses' lived experiences with WPV, their personal feelings about their profession, and the support they received from nursing leadership after WPV occurred. The phenomenological approach describes "things" as they were experienced, such as hearing, seeing, believing, remembering, evaluating, and acting (Polit & Beck, 2021, p. 478). This researcher wanted to explore the problem of WPV from the perspective of those who deal with it most.

Target Population and Sample

The researcher chose a different target population and sample for the research study. This researcher described the sample as persons who were rich in information, allowing the researcher to uncover various realities of nurses' experiences with WPV (Polit & Beck, 2021, p. 497). The researcher then used the study sample to describe the larger nursing population.

Population

For this research study, the larger population considered was registered nurses. The researcher narrowed the target population by including nurses who had experienced WPV from patients, family members, and visitors. The accessible population was the sample of nurses willing to discuss their encounters with WPV (Polit & Beck, 2021). The researcher then used the results to generalize the larger nursing population (Polit & Beck, 2021). This researcher considered assessing a sample size of 15-20 nurses with various experiences of WPV to ensure a representative sample to predict those of the larger population closely. Still, this researcher collected data until saturation (Polit & Beck, 2021).

Sample

This researcher initially used convenience sampling, or "volunteer sampling" (Polit & Beck, 2021, p. 498), by having participants self-identify as nurses who had experienced WPV. Due to the study of a profoundly personal phenomenon, many participants provided sufficient data for the controversial topic of WPV (Polit & Beck, 2021). The researcher also used snowball sampling, "where earlier participants recommended further study participants" who they knew had experienced WPV (Polit & Beck, 2021, p. 498). Purposive sampling, which involved the researcher selecting specific participants that benefited the study, was used to obtain study participants with information-rich experiences of WPV (Polit & Beck, 2021).

Purposive sampling continued until the researcher reached data saturation, meaning the researcher obtained no new information, and redundancy occurred (Polit & Beck, 2021). Polit and Beck (2021, p. 504) noted that phenomenologists "typically rely on small samples, 10-15 participants." Although the participants experienced WPV, the researcher explored the diversity of WPV experienced by each participant. The quality of data obtained also affected the sample size. Participants openly shared various personal experiences of WPV or multiple examples of WPV, which aided the researcher in the richness of data (Polit & Beck, 2021).

Procedures

Terminology must first be understood to replicate a research study. Polit and Beck (2021) reviewed that the research methods should provide other researchers with sufficient detail to replicate the study and elaborate on study design features. In the procedures section, this researcher explained the procedures and instruments used in this study, the rationale for their use, and detailed descriptions of how the researcher's method was carried out (Polit & Beck, 2021).

Participant Selection

This researcher began this qualitative study with a clear idea about the general population of RNs and pursued generalized results (Polit & Beck, 2021). To characterize the accessible population, this researcher used eligibility criteria for study participants (Polit & Beck, 2021). Specific eligibility criteria included nurses who had experienced forms of WPV from their patients, family members, and visitors during their careers. As previously mentioned, the researcher used purposive sampling to estimate a need for 10-15 study participants. However, this researcher collected data until saturation occurred (Polit & Beck, 2021).

This researcher posted a flyer to recruit study participants using social media platforms like Facebook and Instagram. This researcher used a specific email address for this research study to communicate with interested study participants. This researcher sent the informed consent form (ICF) to study participants using this email address to provide additional details and allow them time to prepare questions before the study interview. After signing the ICF, the researcher scheduled a Zoom meeting at the participant's convenience. The Zoom meetings were audio-recorded for the researcher to transcribe verbatim, and the researcher began the semi-structured interview. This researcher offered no monetary incentives for study participation.

Protection of Participants

Polit and Beck (2021) discussed that a fundamental and ethical demand of collecting research with human subjects includes protecting the rights of the research participants. The University of Mount Olive's IRB completed the formal review of this research before this researcher initiated participant recruitment. This researcher asked participants to sign an informed consent form before the interview began that specified the risks of study participation. The informed consent form specified that study participation involved minimal risk, meaning "risks no greater than those encountered in the daily life of routine procedures" (Polit & Beck, 2021, p. 137). The researcher remained sensitive to the potential risks of study participants throughout the study (Polit & Beck, 2021).

The study participants were de-identified, removing information that could reveal their identity in the final study data (Polit & Beck, 2021). The researcher chose to interview participants via the Zoom platform to further protect participants' privacy by not segregating any personal behaviors that may unfold during data collection in a private setting such as a participant's home (Polit & Beck, 2021). This researcher used broad descriptions to identify participants, such as numbers and a generalized description of their work setting (Polit & Beck, 2021). This researcher did not name places of employment, and the researcher used general geographical locations to protect participants' privacy further.

Expert Review

In qualitative studies, using open-ended questions to collect data, statistical validity, and reliability testing cannot be done. Therefore, this researcher discussed their outlook, self-demands, and ingenuity to ensure high-quality research was conducted (Polit & Beck, 2021). This researcher discussed personal qualifications, experience, and the process of reflexive journaling to establish confidence in study findings (Polit & Beck, 2021). The researcher's Master of Science in Nursing (MSN) Faculty Thesis Chair, Dr. Joy Kieffer, later Dr. Nancy Mimm, and the researcher's collaborative mentor, Dr. Mark Hand, provided feedback on interview questions, and the University's IRB approved them.

Data Collection

Each participant contacted the researcher via an email address used for this study to express interest in participating. Furthermore, once the researcher received notification via email, the following occurred (Polit & Beck, 2021):

- This researcher ensured the potential participant met the inclusion eligibility criteria for study participation, encompassing registered nurses who had experienced WPV.
- This researcher sent an informed consent form to the potential participant for extensive review and signature.

- After sending the informed consent form to the participant, this researcher answered all questions satisfactorily, and the informed consent form was signed before the audio-recorded interview. This researcher stored informed consent forms on this researcher's computer per the IRB's policy (UMO IRB Policy and Procedure Manual, 2018, p. 23).
- The participant signed the informed consent form and agreed that study participation was strictly voluntary, without monetary incentive.
- The researcher initiated the audio-recorded interview with participant demographic questions and ice-breaking exchanges to establish rapport (Polit & Beck, 2021).
- The researcher conducted the interviews using semi-structured, open-ended questions.
- The researcher took personal and reflective notes about the researcher's feelings and reflections in a private, audio-recorded reflexive journal, which this researcher will keep for three years per the IRB policy (Polit & Beck, 2021).
- This researcher made additional notes about participant observation to provide a deeper understanding and familiarity with the specific nurse's situation (Polit & Beck, 2021, p. 528; UMO et al. of Policy & Procedure, 2018, p. 23).
- Verbatim transcriptions of the audio-recorded interviews were conducted immediately following the participant's interviews in a Microsoft Word

document. They were sent to the study participants for accuracy review before being used for data analysis (Polit & Beck, 2021).

- This researcher's audio-recorded reflexive journal of participant observation added a richer understanding of human behaviors and situations to provide deeper meanings to specific instances of WPV (Polit & Beck, 2021, p. 528).
- This researcher used bracketing in the researcher's journal, which involved recording the researcher's personal beliefs, opinions, and biases during participant interviews (Polit & Beck, 2021). The researcher's journal will be maintained for three years per the IRB policy (UMO IRB Policy & Procedure Manual, 2018, p. 23).
- This researcher began data analysis, which included coding each participant's interview. Coding was performed by this researcher using a manual method to allow immersion and familiarity with the data (Polit & Beck, 2021).
- This researcher utilized comments and notes in the transcribed Microsoft Word document to highlight specific themes. This researcher coded the initial interview with the MSN Faculty Thesis Chair to ensure the novice researcher's accuracy and understanding of the coding process. This researcher coded the remaining interviews independently.
- This researcher conducted participant interviews until data saturation occurred. Data saturation is "sampling to the point at which no new information is obtained, and redundancy is achieved" (Polit & Beck, 2021,

p. 502). This allowed in-depth data to display patterns, categories, and dimensions of the phenomenon of WPV (Polit & Beck, 2021).

Data Analysis

The qualitative approach to this study created narrative descriptions that depicted experiences of WPV that nurses encountered in the workplace from patients, family members, and visitors. Polit and Beck (2021) explained a manual approach to data analysis, which this researcher used by clustering related types of WPV into schemes. By identifying categories in the transcribed interviews, this researcher identified themes to build an extensive description of nurses' encounters with WPV (Polit & Beck, 2021). The researcher continued interviews until this researcher's coding showed that data was saturated, and no other categories could be obtained (Polit & Beck, 2021).

As Polit and Beck (2021) mentioned, this researcher interpreted each interview exclusively to understand purposeful patterns from participants. This researcher identified themes that contributed to a rich portrayal of the phenomena studied through emerging data patterns (Polit & Beck, 2021). After carefully reviewing each transcription, a specific code and theme were assigned to examples of WPV and placed into a code/frequency table. The themes were color-coded to improve the ease of review for this researcher. This researcher used a code/frequency table to illustrate specific codes for each theme and verbatim illustrations of WPV for themes, with a participant number. By coding the data, this researcher emphasized relevant data that applied to the population of nurses and the specific instances of WPV that were individual to participants (Polit & Beck, 2021). This researcher searched for underlying conceptualizations and strived to understand the broader meanings articulated with data collection (Polit & Beck, 2021).

Instruments

In this section, the researcher clarifies the instruments used to collect data for this qualitative research study. These instruments included this researcher, audio-recorded interviews, and the transcription of interviews in Microsoft Word documents. This section also includes this researcher's role and a description of the semi-structured, open-ended interview questions.

The Role of the Researcher

This researcher conducted audio-recorded, open-ended, semi-structured interviews via Zoom in a private, quiet location. This researcher began the interview with demographic questions about the participant's age, gender, and experience in their respective nursing careers. Polit and Beck (2021, p. 514) highlighted a "topic guide," which ensured this researcher asked participants corresponding questions about WPV experiences, allowing them to reply freely. Questions were structured chronologically from general to more specific, and this researcher also listed probe questions designed to elicit more comprehensive information from participants (Polit & Beck, 2021).

Polit and Beck (2021) described the role of the researcher in qualitative studies as that of the data collection instrument. Still, the researcher is the author of the analytical process, using qualifications, skills, and reflexivity to establish confidence in the study results (Polit & Beck, 2021). This researcher was aware of personal beliefs that could affect the data collection. This researcher is an RN who has had recurrent experience with WPV. This researcher was not in an administrative role with any study participants. This researcher journaled thoughts, opinions, and biases in a private journal that will be maintained per IRB policy for three years after the study's conclusion (UMO IRB Policy & Procedure Manual, 2018, p. 23).

This researcher acquired training for research, ethics, compliance, and safety while conducting research with human subjects through The Collaborative Institutional Training Initiative (CITI Program) and instruction throughout graduate studies at the University of Mount Olive (Collaborative Institutional Training Initiative Program, n.d.). Applying the Polit and Beck (2021) textbook, *Nursing Research: Generating and Assessing Evidence for Nursing Practice*, also offered in-depth training on collecting reliable qualitative data and preparing and conducting semi-structured study interviews (Polit & Beck, 2021). This researcher ensured credibility through verbatim transcriptions of subject interviews and performed the initial coding process with the MSN Faculty Thesis Chair. Additional training included over 11 years of nursing experience in various areas, two national nursing certifications, precepting emergency medical services (EMS) students, paramedics, new graduate nurses, new hires, experienced nurses, and nursing students. This researcher earned a Bachelor of Science in Nursing (BSN) degree from East Carolina University (ECU), which required practical completion of a nursing research course.

Polit and Beck (2021) discussed that this researcher used a private reflexive journal during data collection to address bias and previous familiarity with WPV. This researcher sought to remain unbiased and impartial to create an environment where participants felt at ease freely expressing their experiences of WPV (Polit & Beck, 2021). This researcher used bracketing, "the process of identifying and holding abeyance predetermined views and opinions about the phenomenon under study," to note personal feelings or predispositions during the interview process (Polit & Beck, 2021, p. 478). To remain unbiased, this researcher bracketed in an audio-recorded private journal to separate personal experiences from those of the study participants, and will be kept by this researcher as raw data for three years, per the IRB policy (UMO IRB Policy and Procedure Manual, 2018, p. 23).

Guiding Interview Questions

Using Husserl and Heidegger's approach to phenomenology, this researcher attempted to understand the critical truths about reality in the everyday experiences of RNs who routinely experience WPV (Polit & Beck, 2021). Four aspects of lived experiences interest phenomenologists, including lived space, body, time, and human relation, to give meaning to human existence (Polit & Beck, 2021). This researcher formulated a written guide of semi-structured, open-ended interview questions while encouraging participants to talk liberally about the matters discussed. This researcher asked probing questions to prompt more detailed information on WPV incidences when necessary. The semi-structured, open-ended interview guide consisted of the following questions:

1. Please tell me about yourself. What is your age? Your gender?
2. How long have you worked as a registered nurse?
3. What type of settings have you worked in during your career?

4. What type of setting do you currently work in?
5. What are some experiences you have had with WPV from patients, family members, and visitors? Please give me examples. This question was asked because this researcher wanted to understand the relation to Ida Jean Orlando's nursing process discipline theory (Orlando, 1961, as cited in Petiprin, 2023). This researcher was interested in the initial patient presentation, immediate reactions, the nursing process, and process improvement to reduce instances of WPV (Orlando, 1961, as cited in Petiprin, 2023).
6. How was the instance of violence handled by nursing leadership and management? Please give me examples. This question was asked because this researcher wanted to ascertain if nurses were effectively prepared to meet the needs of patients susceptible to violence in distressing situations and how to mitigate violence when it occurs (Orlando, 1961, as cited in Petiprin, 2023).
7. Please tell me how leadership supported you when you experienced WPV. If you did not feel supported, will you please explain what occurred? This question was asked because Orlando's theory is founded on concepts that incorporate appropriately educating staff on addressing WPV and using process improvement when WPV occurs (Orlando, 1961, as cited in Petiprin, 2023).
8. What is the process to report WPV, and how do you feel that reporting WPV is handled by leadership? Why? This question was asked to understand the

procedure for reporting WPV and to recognize if nurses felt empowered by nursing leadership and management that created a zero-tolerance policy for WPV.

9. How does this make you feel to experience WPV from patients, family members, and visitors? Please give me personal and professional examples. This researcher asked this question to investigate the need for healthcare reform regarding violence against nurses and to explore nurses' occupational commitment (Báez-León et al., 2016; Beattie et al., 2019; Bildik et al., 2022; Dadashzadeh et al., 2019; Doehring et al., 2023; Kiymaz & Koç, 2023; Lim et al., 2022; Moman et al., 2020; Nevels et al., 2020; Ogboghodo & Okojie, 2020).
10. Tell me about times WPV created burnout or feelings of dissatisfaction with your role as a nurse. This question was asked because this researcher wanted to identify how nurses could be further empowered when dealing with cases of WPV. Additionally, this researcher wanted to learn if policies and procedures are failing to safeguard nurses when WPV occurs and if these RNs lacked leadership and management who enforced a zero-tolerance policy of WPV or discouraged reporting incidents of violence (Orlando, 1961, as cited by Petiprin, 2023).
11. Will you please tell me about the adverse ways WPV has affected your ability to provide quality patient care? This researcher wanted to know how nurses handled WPV in distressing situations and whether they could meet the patient's immediate needs (Orlando, 1961, as cited by Petiprin, 2023).

12. If you have ever considered leaving the nursing profession due to WPV from patients, family members, and visitors, will you please tell me about this? The researcher asked this question to understand better the distressing impact WPV has on nurses and provide insight into process improvements for mitigating WPV (Orlando, 1961, as cited by Petiprin, 2023).

Ethical Considerations

Polit and Beck (2021) reviewed the importance of this researcher's obligation to protect the participants throughout the study by maintaining strict data confidentiality. The IRB considered this research exempt because the interviews did not identify the human subjects in any fashion. Polit and Beck (2021, p. 133) stated, "Researchers must avoid, prevent, or minimize harm in research with humans." Study participants made informed and voluntary decisions to participate in the research. They signed an informed consent document agreeing to participation, understanding that they could withdraw participation at any time (UMO IRB Policy and Procedure Manual, 2018, p. 19; Polit & Beck, 2021, p. 134).

Polit and Beck (2021) acknowledged that authors of historical literature perpetrated ethical transgressions against human participants when obtaining research. This researcher did not identify study participants by name, the facilities where they work, or the specific settings in which they were employed (UMO IRB Policy and Procedure Manual, 2018, p. 20). This researcher collected data outside the participant's place of employment, in a private setting, at the participant's convenience. Data and results will be maintained on this researcher's computer without access to others for at least three years per the IRB policy (UMO IRB Policy and Procedure Manual, 2018, p. 23). This researcher ensured the sound construction of the study and the approval from the University of Mount Olive's IRB before the research began (American Nurses Association, 2015; UMO IRB Policy and Procedure Manual, 2018).

Summary

This researcher completed a qualitative research study to explore the lived experiences of acute care nurses who experience workplace violence from patients, family members, and visitors while providing patient care. Semi-structured open-ended interviews were conducted and transcribed verbatim into Microsoft Word. This researcher sent transcribed interviews to study participants via email for review, and read and evaluated each transcription for specific themes and organized codes. This researcher documented the data analysis process in an organized table demonstrating the codes, themes, examples of direct quotes, the frequency of the theme occurring, and the number of participants who explained the various themes in their interviews. The table allowed this researcher to demonstrate complete data saturation and end the data collection process. In Chapter 4, this researcher describes the study's results, the data collected, the results from data analysis, and the findings of this research study.

CHAPTER 4. PRESENTATION OF THE DATA

In Chapter 4, this researcher describes this study's results, presenting the data obtained and analyzed. Polit and Beck (2021) described data analysis as a way for the researcher to organize, provide structure to, and elicit meaning from data. In this chapter, this researcher will introduce the researcher's role, provide greater detail about the study sample, and discuss the research methodology this researcher used to analyze the data.

Introduction: The Study and the Researcher

This researcher is an acute care emergency department nurse with over 11 years of nursing experience in various trauma and emergency department roles for adult and pediatric patients. This researcher was motivated to explore the lived experiences of WPV compared to other nurses due to the ample experience with WPV in the emergency department setting. This researcher's work experience strengthens and limits study objectivity; however, this researcher utilized bracketing to remain unbiased in analyzing the study's data. Polit and Beck (2021, p. 512) stated that researchers should "go native" or avoid becoming overly emotionally involved with participants to ensure they collect meaningful and trustworthy data. This researcher had extensive first-hand knowledge of WPV against nurses in the ED setting; however, this researcher attempted to interview nurses from various backgrounds to provide a clear picture of current WPV trends. To avoid bias, this researcher used reflexive audio-journaling prior to data analysis to be mindful of personal feelings or potential biases. As suggested by Polit and Beck, this researcher used reflexivity to consider this researcher's individual experiences with WPV and remain objective during data collection and analysis.

This researcher first conducted a practice semi-structured interview to ensure that methods, procedures, and interviewing skills were sufficient with the formulated topic guide (Polit & Beck, 2021). This researcher recruited a friend to participate in the practice interview, as they did not meet the study eligibility criteria. This opportunity also allowed this researcher to practice using recording equipment and techniques such as bracketing. As a novice researcher, this practice interview was beneficial in boosting this researcher's self-introductions, interviewing study participants, and responding to participant statements with probing questions. The individual interviewed was not included in the study data, as they did not meet inclusion and exclusion criteria; it was used to assist the researcher with practicing research techniques.

Description of the Sample

Polit and Beck (2021, p. 497) discussed, "A representative sample is desired in qualitative studies to enhance the likelihood that the measurements accurately reflect and can be generalized to the common population." The research sample consisted of seven female participants aged between 27 and 66 (Table 4.1). Five participants worked day shifts, and one strictly worked night shifts. Four participants had a Bachelor of Science in Nursing (BSN) degree, and two had an Associate's Degree in Nursing (ADN).

Two participants were excluded from the data as this researcher could not salvage interview recordings due to computer malfunctions. Although these two participants were willing to re-interview, the researcher and participants' schedules did not align for this to occur. Participants' experience as a registered nurse (RN) ranged from four to 45 years. All six participants were included in the study's data.

There were no withdrawals from the research study. The six participant interviews were all conducted as planned, without disruptions.

TABLE 4.1 PARTICIPANT DEMOGRAPHICS

Participant	Age	Gender	Years of RN Experience	Degree	Current role
1	48	F	23	ADN	Emergency Department
2	32	F	10	BSN	Intravenous (IV) Drip Spa
3	39	F	12	BSN	Stay-at-home mom
4	66	F	45	ADN	Perioperative
5	37	F	13	BSN	Perioperative
6	27	F	4	BSN	Emergency Department

Research Methodology Applied to the Data Analysis

This researcher audio-recorded participant interviews and completed field notes for each study participant (Polit & Beck, 2021). This researcher completed verbatim transcriptions of each participant interview and implemented content validity by emailing each participant a copy of the transcription for review (Polit & Beck, 2021). By thematically organizing participant transcriptions, this researcher revealed underlying concepts and conceptualizations by carefully scrutinizing the raw data (Polit & Beck, 2021). This researcher reviewed transcribed interviews multiple times, identifying all emerging themes from the raw data (Polit & Beck, 2021). Initially, this researcher and the Faculty Thesis Chair co-developed a coding system. This researcher continued data analysis and coding by using a color-coded organization of themes and abbreviated codes, such as SOL NEEDED, for the solutions needed to resolve WPV.

Presentation of Data and Results of the Analysis

This researcher began data analysis by reading and rereading the valid participant transcriptions to break down data into meaningful coding templates (Polit & Beck, 2021). This researcher made ongoing modifications to accommodate the data as new themes emerged during data analysis (Polit & Beck, 2021). This researcher categorized thirty themes from the raw data obtained through participant interviews. This researcher could not generate new themes after data analysis of six participant interviews (Polit & Beck, 2021). This researcher corroborated data saturation after six participant interviews, confirming that a detailed and thorough description of the phenomenon of WPV against nurses had been achieved (Polit & Beck, 2021).

TABLE 4.2 CODE/FREQUENCY TABLE

Code	Theme	Frequency	Number of Participants	Example Quotes
NEG EMOT	Negative= Feelings of helplessness/defeat	154	6	"...I went back into our lounge and burst into tears..."
EX	Example of WPV	94	6	"...She slapped it out of my hand..."
SOL NEEDED	Negative= A solution is needed to resolve WPV	84	4	"... At the time, there was no standard way to report this..."
NEG LEAD	Negative = Nothing from Leadership	75	6	"The thing that I remember the most was that my charge nurse did not take this patient for me..."
NEG AFF	Negative= Negatively affecting patient care	41	5	"... Hey, charge nurse, can you take this patient..."

NEG RN PROCESS	Negative = The RN does not know what to do with the WPV experience	39	6	"... Until they are right into it, you do not see what is happening..."
SA	Negative= Substance abuse	29	3	"... Patients who take recreational drugs like marijuana, they wake up more confused..."
POS LEAD	Positive = leadership support for WPV	23	5	"...You would call the charge nurse..."
STRESS SIT	Negative= A stressful situation for families	12	1	"... Obviously, it is a very stressful situation for them..."
COWKR SUPPT	Positive= had help and support of colleagues	9	4	"... There are a lot of male nurses who will come in and help..."
MOVE ON	Negative= Having thoughts about moving on from my current role	9	3	"... Yes. It definitely made me burned out..."
POL ASST	Positive= Police assisted Nurses	8	4	"...You have police officers for security..."
POS ADMIN IMPL	Positive = Administrative Implementation of help	8	3	"...So, we actually had the employee assistance program (EAP) coming around onto the unit..."
REST	Negative= Restraint of the patient due to violence	8	3	"...We had to sedate and restrain him..."
POS LAW	Positive = Assault RN has a law	8	1	"...I know that New York State was one of the first states to take that more seriously..."
CAUT	Neutral = More cautious of patient interactions	6	2	"... I am a lot more cautious now..."
INT	Negative= Intimidated by patient	6	2	"...He was scary, he was very intimidating..."
NEG LAW	Negative = Assault RN law does not exist	5	2	"...At that point, assaulting a nurse was not yet a felony..."

LOVE RN	Positive= Love nursing role	5	2	"...I have never considered doing anything else..."
VISIT HRS	Negative= Visiting policy of hospital affecting RN	5	1	"...There have been no visiting hours; they can come and go as they please..."
HI ACUITY	Neutral= Caring for high acuity level patients	4	1	"...High-acuity, very sick patients..."
POS RN PROCESS	Positive= Process that helps nurses mitigate WPV	4	1	"... He started to get used to me, and I am not a violent person at all..."
NOT AFF	Neutral= It did not affect nursing care	3	2	"...I do not really feel like it is affecting my nursing care..."
ANG	Negative= Feelings of anger due to WPV	3	2	"... She got kicked in the head, which made her mad..."
PSYCH PT	Negative= WPV experience with mental health patients	3	2	"...It was one of the psychiatric patients there..."
DEVAL RN	Negative= Nurses are not valued	3	1	"...Actions are not following through on that..."
POS EMOT	Positive= Feelings of support were given	2	2	"...I ended up calling my brother..."
TOUGH	Negative= Experiences of WPV made RNs tougher individuals	1	1	"...The NICU in itself, as any nursing unit, has stresses of its own..."
VAL RN	Positive= Value nurses	1	1	"...People say they value nurses as a profession..."
LEG NEEDED	Negative= Legislation needed to decrease WPV	1	1	"... It is going to come down to legislation..."
MD DIFF	Positive= Doctors attempting to diffuse situations of WPV	1	1	"... It is not until the doctor himself comes out and chastises the patient for their behavior, telling them

				they have to reschedule…”

The top 16 themes that emerged during this study were combined into four common categories. Six themes combined in “Things Nurses Experience” include negative emotions such as helplessness and defeat, and a solution is needed to resolve workplace violence (WPV). These things negatively affect patient care: the RN does not know what to do with the WPV experience, the RN has thoughts of moving on from their current role, and the RN is more cautious of patient interactions. Four themes combined in “Healthcare System Defeat” are examples of workplace violence, no assistance or support from leadership, substance abuse, and stressful situations for families. Three themes combined in “Working as a Team” include Leadership support for WPV, help and support from colleagues, and nurses' assistance from police. Three themes combined in “Support for Nurses” include restraint of the patient due to violence, administrative implementation of help, and laws against assaulting healthcare workers.

Things Nurses Experience

In this study, participants frequently mentioned negative emotions (NEG EMOT), such as feelings of hopelessness and defeat (154 times) due to experiences with WPV. Participant One discussed a pediatric patient who created a weapon out of a toothbrush and stated, “You know this is the thought that keeps coming back; this is not what I signed up for.” Participant Two described her time working at an inner-city, level-one trauma center and expressed, “I guess… I was so young, I was 23 back then, and I was kind of like, this is what nurses do. This is just what happens if you are going to work at a place like this." Doehring et al. (2023) explained that violence in healthcare increases the risk of burnout, PTSD, decreased job satisfaction, and feelings of avoidance and futility. Most participants expressed these feelings in detail throughout their interviews.

Participants explained 41 instances in which WPV had negatively affected (NEG AFF) patient care. Participant Six described that those violent patients took time away from providing patient care to others and performing routine nursing duties like passing daily medications. Participant Six stated, "It was not just affecting us as nurses; it was affecting our other patients, too." Participant Six also mentioned, "You feel helpless because our other patients who are alert and oriented would come and say, I am scared. What if that person comes into my room tonight?" Participant One explained that they did not feel that WPV affected their nursing care; however, "I do find that I lose my temper with these kids a little bit more." Dafny and Beccaria (2020) considered WPV towards healthcare workers (HCWs) who experience violence almost daily, feel it is a routine part of their jobs, and feel a burden to accept violence due to a culture in healthcare that makes violence challenging to address.

Participants expressed negative feelings about not knowing how to handle WPV or what to do when it occurs (NEG RN PROCESS) 39 times throughout the study interviews. Participant Three recalled past instances of verbal violence, aggression, and passive-aggressive communication. Participant Three stated, "It was just accepted. It was something you had to learn to deal with... It did not feel like anybody else thought anything of it as a new nurse. It was just tolerated." Participant Two recalled, "Back then, it was just accepted, but it probably took me a few years to realize that there were other outlets and things in nursing that I should consider to get away from those things." Doehring et al. (2023) reported that WPV against HCWs was expected, with abusive events occurring almost daily, with up to 20% of events involving physical violence.

Study participants discussed their thoughts about moving on from their current role (MOVE ON) nine times as a nurse due to WPV. Participant Two recollected, "I would say I have considered leaving nursing due to what nursing is as a whole." Participant Two also stated, "... you can only take so much." Participant Three recently left their career as a full-time RN to rear young children. Participant Three said, "At this point in time, just thinking on a future date of me returning to nursing, that is not in my plan in the near future." Additionally, Participant Two mentioned, "...I just felt very burned out at the end. I loved what I did, and I never saw myself in any other role in the nursing field, but I was just very burned out...". Participant Four explained, "I kind of got burned out with that high stress and just went out and did agency work." This researcher discussed their intent to leave their RN role. Participant Six recalled, "... I don't have that perspective", as they discussed not experiencing routine WPV. Kiymaz & Koç (2023, p. 766) concerned, "Factors related to the organizational structure, such as the physical conditions in the place of work and job security, may directly affect an employee's intention to resign."

Two participants mentioned being more cautious of patient interactions (CAUT) six times throughout the study. Participant One stated, "I feel like I am a lot more hesitant, which is a new feeling for me... I am usually pretty confident in my dealings with patients...". Participant Two described their work at an inner-city Level I trauma center. They explained, "...how do you keep nurses in these roles that are experienced and really able to provide top-notch, quality care to get good patient outcomes in this type of environment?". Kiymaz and Koç (2023) discussed the need for nurses' working conditions to be improved with a decreased workload to maximize occupational commitment and reduce their intent to resign.

Healthcare System Defeat

The Joint Commission (2023a) created a Workplace Violence Prevention Compendium of Resources document that became effective on 1/1/2022. Unfortunately, this researcher uncovered 94 instances of workplace violence (EX) throughout six study participant interviews. Participant Four explained, "Most of the time, it is verbal abuse... They can get pretty mouthy and belligerent verbally." Participant Five discussed a patient for whom she accepted a bedside shift report, stating, "A patient was totally upset with how his doctors were communicating with him about what was going on with his care. He was super upset, first kind of ignoring me, and then verbally aggressive with me." Participant Six described navigating difficult conversations with a patient's aggressive family member. Participant Six recalled, "She would get very angry about everything we had done wrong...". Participant Two described a mental health patient and said, "... I remember he was trying to grab the women walking by him... he was trying to stick his arms on women's groin area." Participant One described an incident with a patient's father who became irate about end-of-life care, remembering, "... He threatened to kill me." Workplace violence (WPV) is an ongoing global problem, and extensive literature and many studies continue to examine ways to mitigate and end violence in the healthcare arena (Báez-León et al., 2016; Beattie et al., 2019; Bildik et al., 2022; Dadashzadeh et al., 2019; Doehring et al., 2023; Kiymaz & Koç, 2023; Lim et al., 2022; Moman et al., 2020; Nevels et al., 2020; Ogboghodo & Okojie, 2020).

This researcher learned that all six study participants experienced 75 instances where they did not receive support from leadership (NEGLEAD). Participant Four described being kicked in the chest by a cardiac intensive care unit (ICU) patient. Participant Four further explained what nursing leadership did; she stated, "Well, nothing really... We had to write the incident report... but never really had any management input... or anything else to try to prevent future things from happening." Participant Five asked leadership for assistance with changing assignments and reported, "They do not really want to do anything... There has to be a valid reason someone is asking for a change." Participant Three explained that when requesting leadership support while dealing with WPV, "It was rare that they would actually ever be removed." Báez-León et al. (2016, p. 363) mentioned, "Rather, participants' appraisal of the situation as involving little or no costs in relation to benefits appears to be a critical factor when it comes to helping victims."

Colvonen et al. (2019) explained that substance abuse disorders are often a means to cope with anxiety, pain, and insomnia. Three participants mentioned substance abuse disorders (SA) 29 times throughout this study. Participant Four stated, "They are not always truthful about how much they have been drinking. I have also had patients who come into the ER freaking out from their drug and cocaine use." Participant Three explained she did not encounter many violent mothers in the neonatal intensive care unit (NICU); however, "many moms who were just strung out." Additionally, Participant Three recalled parents who, "The mom and dad were both substance users... he was just paranoid... he was just very belligerent... you could not reason with him."

During her interview, one participant discussed 12 stressful situations for families (STRESS SIT). Participant Three stated, "Obviously, it is a very stressful situation for them, and a lot of the population that we serve are people who just have poor coping skills. So put in a stressful situation, that is a recipe for just some craziness..." Additionally, Participant Three mentioned a mother present for her infant's NICU stay, "... she just had to be there when anybody was doing anything to her. I mean, stand over you when you were doing anything... question what you were doing."

Working As a Team

Five participants discussed 23 examples of positive leadership when supporting nurses affected by WPV (POS LEAD). Participant One explained, "... we actually had the employee assistance program (EAP) coming around onto the unit... I got to spend some time in a session with the EAP...". Participant One expressed gratitude with leadership "... calling the police and making sure the situation is as under control as it can be." "Participant Four recalled positive leadership after an incident with WPV, stating, "I went to another area of that ICU... so I worked in a different pod that night...".

Four participants described nine instances of having the support and help of their colleagues (COWKR SUPPT) when they experienced WPV. Participant Two described acute psychiatric patients in the ED. They explained, "I feel like at the moment you have support in places like that because you have police officers for security, and there are a lot of male nurses there who will come in and help physically in the acute phase." Participant Six stated, "My experienced co-workers and I can usually talk about it and say oh, that was just a thing that happened, and we can move on."

Four participants mentioned eight times that police assisted nurses (POL ASST) with WPV. Participant Two explained, "... you have support in places like that because you have police officers for security...". Participant One described police assistance when a mental health patient in the ED created a weapon from a toothbrush. Participant One stated, "... we ended up having to call the police for that situation. They ended up tackling him to the ground, he got restrained, and just some of the things that he said to me...".

Support for Nurses

Muir-Cochrane et al. (2020) explained that restraints are used to control and protect violent patients and staff and are to be utilized only as a last resort when all behavioral modification alternatives have been exhausted. Among participants, the use of restraints due to violence (REST) was mentioned eight times throughout the interviews. Participant Two described a patient, "He had to be restrained, again, because he could not control himself." Participant Two also recalled a patient who kicked her in the chest and kicked a colleague in the head. Participant Two stated, "We had to have help to restrain her because she could not control her behavior, and I do not think she was in her right mind." Participant One described an event that led her to tears, "... we had to sedate and restrain him. I went back into our lounge and just burst into tears because I did not know what to do. I did not know how to process that...".

Positive implementation of help from leadership (POS ADMIN IMPL) was mentioned eight times among study participants. Participant Five recalled her experience and said, "I feel that in the few years, I have worked for a certain company, they are more aware of WPV, and there is a more strategic chain of command where you go to report things... in a couple of years I have been here they found that WPV is something that happens to a lot of nurses...". Additionally Participant Five mentioned, "... They are actually mandating a lot of this education. So, I do feel like it is getting better." Participant Six described her leadership as positive, "... we could always email or call my boss, and she would be very helpful, and work through it, discuss what happened, and what we could do to make it better. She was very empowering."

Participants mentioned the benefits of a law against assaulting nurses (POS LAW) eight times. Participant One explained, "I know New York state was one of the first states to make that more serious, but even at that point, we were not quite there yet...". Participant Two remembered changes in healthcare safety laws and said, "It was not in place yet. I think it came into place either while I was there or right after I left the new law that supposedly makes it a harsher punishment for assaulting healthcare workers." McKay et al. (2020) described violence against healthcare workers (HCWs) as an unchanged global phenomenon. McKay et al. explained that government officials must take immediate action against WPV against healthcare workers. Implementing legislation with strict punishment against perpetrators of violence is a positive solution geared toward combating WPV in the healthcare arena.

The two participants with the highest occurrences of WPV were currently practicing nursing in the ED and perioperative settings, respectively. Sachdeva et al. (2019) explained that studies had identified EDs as high-risk settings for WPV against healthcare workers. Doehring et al. (2023) reported that WPV in healthcare is commonplace; however, it may be more abundant in the ED setting.

Doehring et al. (2023) also expressed that while approximately one in 275 ED patients become violent during their ED visit, violence directed at healthcare workers frequently goes underreported and unreported to nurses' employers. Doehring et al. incorporated reasons for underreporting and underreporting of WPV, incorporating time constraints in a busy ED, fear of patient retaliation, loss of anonymity, and lack of confidence in nursing leadership that corrective actions against perpetrators of WPV would result. Nevels et al. (2020) defended that understanding employee vulnerabilities improves safety for healthcare workers experiencing WPV. According to Nevels et al., victims who experienced trauma related to WPV included the following: 70% were female, 67% were aged 25-54, 70% worked in the healthcare or social services settings, 21% required three or more days away from work to recover, and 19% required three to five days away from work.

Participants who expressed the most frequent occurrences of receiving no support from nursing leadership had the following work experience listed in descending order by primary nursing specialty. Participant Six experienced the most significant lack of leadership support and practice in med-surg, rehabilitation, and ED nursing settings. A perioperative nurse followed this participant, followed by a med-surg and perioperative nurse, followed by a NICU nurse, and lastly, two ED nurses. Doehring et al. (2023, p. 3) stated, "In the current environment of staffing shortages, retention challenges, and recruitment difficulties, decreasing workplace abuse of staff should be considered an essential part of a strategy to retain experienced and qualified healthcare workers." Doehring et al. also indicated that few studies are available to evaluate organizational or environmental interventions in healthcare that target reductions in WPV, and this area warrants further investigation.

While assessing the departments' socio-demographic characteristics and working conditions, Bildik et al. (2022) examined the relationship between safety and staff's perception of safety in emergency departments. Bildik et al. mentioned that while WPV is an old, chronic problem, awareness of it is increasing daily due to the alarming rates at which healthcare workers suffer WPV despite increased precautions and the pursuit of legal measures.

Participant Three, who practiced nursing in the NICU, expressed experiencing the most significant occurrences of feeling helpless and defeated. The following participants with the highest events of helplessness and defeat included the subsequent participants: Participant Six, with med-surg/rehabilitation/ED nursing experience; Participant Four, with primarily perioperative experience; Participant One, mainly an ED nurse; Participant Two, specifically an ED nurse; lastly, Participant Five, primarily a med-surg and perioperative nurse.

Bildik et al. (2022) mentioned that violence affects all areas of life, with 1.3 million deaths annually attributed to violence. The United States Department of Labor (n.d.) explained that when Congress passed the Occupational Safety and Health Act of 1970, the Occupational Safety and Health Administration (OSHA) was created to ensure safe and healthful working conditions for individuals by setting and enforcing standards and providing training, education, and assistance. As rates of WPV in healthcare continue at staggering levels, OSHA and global, national, state, and local organizations seek viable solutions to mitigate WPV in healthcare.

Summary

This researcher revealed the top themes from the semi-structured interview questions with the six study participants in Chapter Four. Unfortunately, authors of the current literature surrounding WPV highlighted many of the recurrent themes for the nursing profession that were identified by this researcher (Báez-León et al., 2016; Beattie et al., 2019; Bildik et al., 2022; Dadashzadeh et al., 2019; Doehring et al., 2023; Kiymaz & Koç, 2023; Lim et al., 2022; Moman et al., 2020; Nevels et al., 2020; Ogboghodo & Okojie, 2020). Nurse satisfaction, retention, and professional commitment are all affected by many of the problems studied in this researcher's master's thesis. In Chapter Five, this researcher will discuss the meaning of the themes and clusters that emerged during the data analysis process in greater detail.

CHAPTER 5. DISCUSSION, IMPLICATIONS, RECOMMENDATIONS

Chapter 5 of the thesis discusses how the researcher answered the research question and its potential implications for nursing. The researcher also mentioned previous literature and broader communities of interest. The introductory qualitative study aimed to explore the lived experiences of acute care nurses who had experienced workplace violence (WPV) from patients, visitors, and family members, and the study results were presented objectively in the previous chapters. However, in this chapter, the researcher will describe the evaluation and utilization of study data. The study results provide helpful information for future studies on WPV in healthcare.

Summary of the Results

The prevalence of workplace violence (WPV) in the healthcare sector is a global concern. Despite numerous policies and regulations, WPV continues to occur, with 75% of incidents occurring in healthcare and social service settings. This issue is not limited to a specific region or country; current management strategies have proven ineffective. Several studies, including those by Báez-León et al. (2016), Beattie et al. (2019), Bildik et al. (2022), Dadashzadeh et al. (2019), Doehring et al. (2023), Kiymaz & Koç (2023), Lim et al. (2022), Moman et al. (2020), Nevels et al. (2020), and Ogboghodo & Okojie (2020), have highlighted the need for further research and improved measures to prevent WPV in the healthcare setting.

The supporting literature spanned globally, including Spain (Báez-León et al., 2016), Australia (Beattie et al., 2019), the U.S. (Bildik et al., 2022; Doehring et al., 2023; Moman et al., 2020; Nevels et al., 2020), Iran (Dadashzadeh et al., 2019), Turkey (Kiymaz & Koç, 2023), Malaysia (Lim et al., 2022), and Nigeria (Ogboghodo &

Okojie, 2020). National and state nurses' associations (American Nurses Association, 2015; Emergency Nurses Association, 2023; National Council of State Boards of Nursing, 2023; North Carolina Board of Nursing, 2023), government organizations (The Joint Commission, 18 June 2021; 2023a; 2023b; United States Department of Labor, n.d.), research, and nursing textbooks (Polit & Beck, 2021; Roush, 2019) provided additional guidance throughout the research process.

This qualitative research study used a descriptive phenomenological approach, which involved semi-structured interviews with registered nurses who had experienced WPV in healthcare. This small exploratory study evaluates nurses' experiences throughout the United States regarding the impacts of WPV, job satisfaction, job retention, and intention to resign. The data from verbatim interview transcriptions was manually analyzed and organized into thematic groupings. This analysis revealed thirty-one themes, with all six participants expressing four common themes: negative emotions, examples of workplace violence, negative leadership, and negative nursing processes. The study's results, which can be generalized to other healthcare settings, can potentially ignite further motivation for future studies based on these findings.

Discussion of the Results

During the interviews with six participants, the most common theme that emerged was the feeling of helplessness and defeat due to workplace violence (WPV). The participants mentioned this theme 154 times, indicating the significant negative impact of WPV on registered nurses. The interviews also revealed that nurses often feel helpless in the face of WPV and cited examples of violent patient encounters 94 times. These findings are alarming and highlight the urgent need for measures to address workplace violence in the healthcare industry.

Participant One depicted a belligerent father whose son recently underwent surgery, stating, "This is your fault. You did this, you know, that tube needs to be out; what did you do?" Participant One went on to describe verbal aggression and homicidal threats from the patient's father, who was irate after his child was reintubated following an episode of respiratory decompensation post-operatively. Participant Two portrayed a patient treated in an urban emergency department for substance abuse, reporting, "She was just being super violent, hitting, kicking, and scratching." Participant Three discussed a neonatal intensive care unit (NICU) patient's mother, stating, "This mother who umm... I mean, she was not physically violent or anything like that, but she was just very verbally abusive to the nurses." Participant Four explained, "They can get pretty mouthy and belligerent verbally." Participant Five illustrated a cardiac intensive care unit (ICU) patient who kicked her, stating, "He had me pinned against his bed and the wall. He got himself up and was able to kick. We were trying to hold him down because he had a fresh open chest, and we did not want him to strain himself, but he kicked me in the face." Participant Six portrayed dementia patients in skilled nursing facilities, reporting, "I have had them start to get a little crazy, where they might be lunging or trying to attack...".

Conclusions Based on the Results

The previous section of this thesis focused on the findings of this study. The upcoming section will focus on prior literature and the broader field of interest. The research outcomes were in line with prior studies, and regrettably, the resolution to WPV (workplace violence) is still ongoing.

Comparison of Findings with Theoretical Framework and Previous Literature

The top three themes in this study correspond with the literature in Chapter Two of this thesis. Lim et al. (2022) described the ongoing concern to the public and occupational health sectors due to increasing instances of WPV. Additionally, Lim et al. commented on the negative implications of WPV in healthcare and how it affects the delivery of care, decreases the quality of care, increases missed work days, and many healthcare workers leave their respective fields due to violence.

Feelings of helplessness/hopelessness (NEG EMOT) were discussed the most frequently in study interviews, 154 times, comprising 24% of emerging themes. Interviews identified WPV examples (EX) 94 times, encompassing 14% of the themes discussed. The third most frequently mentioned theme was needing a solution to resolve WPV (SOL NEEDED), identified 84 times, or 13% of the themes mentioned. Nothing from leadership (NEG LEAD) was mentioned 75 times, WPV negatively affecting patient care (NEG AFF) was mentioned 41 times, nurses not knowing what to do with WPV experiences (NEG RN PROCESS) was mentioned 39 times, substance abuse (S.A.) mentioned 29 times, leadership support for WPV (POS LEAD) mentioned 23 times, in totality were discussed 209 times, comprising 32% of interview responses.

The nursing process discipline theory developed by Ida Jean Orlando emphasizes the significance of nurses tending to the immediate needs of patients, even when their behaviors are incongruent or inappropriate (Orlando, 1961, as cited in Petiprin, 2023). In the study, all six participants shared their passion for serving others but also expressed the mental, physical, and emotional challenges associated with frequent encounters with workplace violence (WPV).

Interpretation of the Findings

The study effectively answered the research question on the lived experiences of nurses who have experienced WPV. However, the results were both enlightening and disheartening, revealing that nurses across all healthcare sectors often encounter WPV and feel unsupported by leadership, healthcare policies, and regulations. The findings revealed alarming levels of professional dissatisfaction, violence that affects patient care, feelings of intimidation, devaluation, burnout, and helplessness. One participant even left the healthcare profession entirely. At the same time, several registered nurses reported leaving their previous nursing positions due to the ineffective strategies and policies for mitigating WPV.

A more substantial research question could examine the relationship between instances of WPV, leadership involvement in WPV, and staff turnover. The increased instances of WPV are likely because the nurses interviewed for this study worked in high-acuity areas such as ICUs, E.D.s, and perioperative settings. According to Nevels et al. (2020), healthcare professionals have normalized the occurrence of WPV due to its frequent occurrences. This disappointing reality was abundantly evident among all six study participants.

Several nurses have reported the need for additional staffing to handle violent situations when patients become unmanageable. Research has indicated that WPV is a complex problem requiring immediate intervention worldwide. Many studies have focused on this issue, including Báez-León et al. (2016), Beattie et al. (2019), Bildik et al. (2022), Dadashzadeh et al. (2019), Doehring et al. (2023), Kiymaz & Koç (2023), Lim et al. (2022), Moman et al. (2020), Nevels et al. (2020), and Ogboghodo & Okojie (2020). Furthermore, Kiymaz and Koç (2023) have identified job dissatisfaction as the most significant predictor of nurses' resigning intentions. Future studies may explore the relationship between WPV, strategies to address it, and nurses' resignation intentions and actions.

Limitations

Chapter One of this thesis explains that every study has some realistic limitations. Qualitative studies are no exception, and these limitations may include small sample sizes, limited generalizability of results, idiosyncratic conclusions, and the subjectivity of humans who are fallible research tools (Polit & Beck, 2021). In this study, data collection continued until the point of meeting saturation to understand the abstract phenomena of WPV (Polit & Beck, 2021). The study included six nurse interviews, but a more extensive and diverse group of participants may have provided more substantial study results. Additionally, nurses from other healthcare settings may have provided different information.

The study involved six participants, four of whom had a Bachelor of Science degree in Nursing (BSN), while the remaining two held an Associate's degree in Nursing (ADN). Interviewing a more diverse group of nurses with various education and work experiences may improve the accuracy of study results. According to Polit and Beck (2021), the interpretive phenomenology process involves immersing oneself in another person's world and interpreting their practical understanding, wisdom, and possibilities.

Implications of the Study

The study's implications are significant for nursing theory, the knowledge base of the nursing profession, and the practical applications of nursing policy, procedure, and evidence-based practice (EBP). According to Doehring et al. (2023), WPV is an underreported issue attributed to a lack of policies, cumbersome reporting methods, victim-blaming, and a lack of productive action following violent incidents. Doehring et al. also discussed how WPV often leads to burnout, PTSD, decreased job satisfaction, hyper-alertness, avoidance, and futility, which are common among registered nursing professionals who experience WPV.

Implications for Practice

According to Lim et al. (2022), when acts of WPV occur, healthcare workers may choose to leave their jobs, which can affect the delivery of healthcare services. Moreover, Lim et al. stated that WPV can lead to unequal access to primary healthcare due to increased demand for population health needs. Doehring et al. (2023) found that 63% of emergency department staff feel unsafe at work. Nurses, who spend the most time providing direct patient care, are frequently the target of aggression and violence by patients, visitors, and family members, as reported by Doehring et al. (2023).

Implications for Theory

The theoretical framework used for the foundation of this thesis was Ida Jean Orlando's nursing process discipline theory. All six participants interviewed explained the significance of identifying patient needs despite incongruent behaviors and verbal or physical violence. Participants explained feelings of discouragement, helplessness, and hopelessness when unable to identify the dissatisfaction of their patients. Participant Five described receiving her oncoming shift report on a patient who was verbally aggressive due to communication barriers with the treatment team prior to her assuming care. Participant Five stated, "I just remember it made me feel really upset... I do not think I can help him... I do not think I am the person that can do anything for him...".

In a citation by Petiprin in 2023, Orlando (1961) noted that patient behaviors are often inappropriate and used as a cry for help, requiring nursing intervention. Furthermore, inappropriate patient behaviors frequently improve with nursing intervention. Báez-León et al. (2016) discussed that workplace violence (WPV) often occurs in individuals in stressful situations with poor prognoses. They emphasized the importance of nursing staff understanding the code of conduct to address inappropriate behavior. Báez-León et al. also highlighted the significance of adequate staffing ratios to ensure the safety of staff and patients in healthcare.

Recommendations for Further Research

Doehring et al. (2023) declared WPV a substantial problem affecting RN feelings of burnout and attrition, increasing staffing shortages, recruiting difficulties, and staff retention challenges. This researcher feels that it is necessary to identify policy breakdown that fails to protect staff from WPV and fails to support staff after violence has occurred. Additionally, further research on the relationship between nurses' intention to resign due to WPV by acute care departments would help identify areas that most need policy reform. Further research to investigate the plans of professional and governmental agencies to monetarily contribute to combating WPV would help project potential resources to allocate towards WPV reduction and staff safety.

WPV has numerous adverse effects on healthcare delivery, staff mental and emotional wellness, and the ability to staff the healthcare industry adequately. The key players in the healthcare industry are essential for successful healthcare delivery to patients. In 2023, Kiymaz and Koç noted that nurses' intentions of voluntary resignation were due to dissatisfaction with organizational structure, environmental factors, and the safety conditions of employment, which are critical indicators for job resignation. They also described that occupational commitment to nursing decreases with exposure to WPV. In 2020, Nevels et al. explained that the employer has a moral obligation to provide a safe work environment, and the direct cost of overall injuries and fatalities due to WPV are drivers for a healthcare culture change.

Nevels et al. (2020) described a zero-tolerance policy for WPV, including staff training to help registered nurses mitigate WPV. Additionally, Nevels et al. discussed key prevention tactics, risk-reduction measures, and on-the-job training to ensure the safety of healthcare staff when faced with violence daily. While OSHA has mandated a federal WPV prevention standard, successfully combatting WPV in healthcare requires regulatory compliance, facility support, leadership, and funding.

Conclusion

The study has addressed the issue of nurses' experiences with WPV. However, it has raised further questions about the effectiveness of current strategies. How can nursing administration protect their staff from WPV? Why are quality indicators and WPV rates not enough to drive change when implementing safety measures in healthcare? By combining the literature cited in this study with additional research, nursing leadership can adjust staffing by experience levels, workload, and safety measures to mitigate violence further.

Ongoing challenges with quality care delivery, access to healthcare, and adverse events will continue to increase as the battle against WPV continues. Although eliminating WPV in healthcare is next to impossible, implementing control measures should assist in protecting the staff caring for patients within an organization (Nevels et al., 2023). Although hospitals must meet acceptable standards on Hospital Consumer Assessment of Healthcare Providers and Systems (HCAHPS) surveys to receive federal funding, these reports have been counterproductive in protecting employees against WPV protection. Using the supporting literature (Báez-León et al., 2016; Beattie et al., 2019; Bildik et al., 2022; Dadashzadeh et al., 2019; Doehring et al., 2023; Kiymaz & Koç, 2023; Lim et al., 2022; Moman et al., 2020; Nevels et al., 2020; Ogboghodo & Okojie, 2020), and research findings, nursing administrators, directors, charge nurses, and hospital executives could begin implementing stricter policies against WPV, unit training, and address unit staffing issues to protect patients and staff adequately against violence. Nevels et al. described the need for a multi-prong approach in combating WPV in healthcare. WPV will be an ongoing global healthcare issue without adequate support, funding, and administration tenacity for violence prevention.

REFERENCES

American Nurses Association. (2015). *Code of ethics for nurses with interpretive statements*. American Nurses Publishing.

Báez-León, C., Moreno-Jiménez, B., Aguirre-Camacho, A., & Olmos, R. (2016). Factors influencing intention to help and helping behavior in witnesses of bullying in nursing settings. *Nursing Inquiry*, *23*(4), 358-367. https://doi.org/10.1111/nin.12149

Beattie, J., Griffiths, D., Innes, K., & Morphet, J. (2019). Workplace violence perpetrated by clients of health care: A need for safety and trauma-informed care. *Journal of Clinical Nursing*, *28*(1-2), 116-124. https://doi.org/10.1111/jocn.14683

Bildik, B., Atis, S. E., Cekmen, B., & Dorter, M. (2022). Do we feel safe and confident about workplace violence in the emergency departments? *American Journal of Emergency Medicine*, *59*, 9-14. https://doi.org/10.1016/j.ajem.2022.06.040

Collaborative Institutional Training Initiative Program. (n.d.). *The trusted standard in research, ethics, compliance, and safety training*. CITI Program. Retrieved on March 16, 2023, from https://about.citiprogram.org/

Colvonen, P. J., Ellison, J., Haller, M., & Norman, S. B. (2019). Examining insomnia and PTSD over time in veterans in residential treatment for substance use disorders and PTSD. *Behavioral Sleep Medicine*, *17*(4), 524-535. https://doi.org/10.1080/15402002.2018.1425869

Dadashzadeh, A., Rahmani, A., Hassankhani, H., Boyle, M., Mohammadi, E., & Campbell, S. (2019). Iranian pre-hospital emergency care nurses' strategies to manage workplace violence: A descriptive qualitative study. *Journal of Nursing Management*, *27*(6), 1190-1199. https://doi.org/10.1111/jonm.12791

Dafny, H. A., & Beccaria, G. (2020). I do not even tell my partner: Nurses' perceptions of verbal and physical violence against nurses working in a regional hospital. *Journal of Clinical Nursing*, *29*(17-18), 3336-3348. https://doi.org/10.1111/jocn.15362

Doehring, M. C., Curtice, H., Hunter, B. R., Oaxaca, D. M., Satorius, A., Reed, K., Beckman, A., Vaughn, T., & Palmer, M. (2023). Exploring verbal and physical workplace violence in a large, urban emergency department. *American Journal of Emergency Medicine*, *67*, 1-4. https://doi.org/10.1016/j.ajem.2023.01.036

Emergency Nurses Association. (2023). *Workplace violence*. https://www.ena.org/quality-and-safety/workplace-violence

Felitti, V. J., Anda, R. F., Nordenberg, D., Williamson, D. F., Spitz, A. M., Edwards, V., ... Marks, J. S. (1998). Relationship of childhood abuse and household dysfunction to many of the leading causes of death in adults. The Adverse Childhood Experiences (ACE) study. *American Journal of Preventive Medicine*, *14*(4), 245-258. https://doi.org/10.1016/s0749-3797(98)00017-8

Forkey, H., Gillespie, R. J., Pettersen, T., Lisa Spector, L. S., & Stirling, J. (2014). *Adverse childhood experiences and the lifelong consequences of trauma*. Retrieved July 29, 2023, from https://downloads.aap.org/AAP/PDF/ttb_aces_consequences.pdf

H1. (2023). *Acute care hospitals and their role in healthcare*. https://h1.co/blog/acute-care-hospitals-their-role-in-healthcare/

Kiymaz, D., & Koç, Z. (2023). Workplace violence, occupational commitment, and intention among emergency room nurses: A mixed-methods study. *Journal of Clinical Nursing*, *32*(5-6), 764-779. https://doi.org/10.1111/jocn16331

Lim, M. C., Jeffree, M. S., Saupin, S. S., Giloi, N., & Lukman, K. A. (2022). Workplace violence in healthcare settings: The risk factors, implications, and collaborative preventive measures. *Annals of Medicine and Surgery*, *78*. https://doi.org/10.1016/j.amsu.2022.103727

McKay, D., Heisler, M., Mishori, R., Catton, H., & Kloiber, O. (2020). Attacks against healthcare personnel must stop, especially as the world fights COVID-19. *The Lancet*, *395*(10239), 1743-1745. https://doi.org/10.1016/S0140-6736(20)31191-0

Moman, R. N., Maher, D. P., & Hooten, W. M. (2020). Workplace violence in the setting of pain management. *Mayo Clinic Proceedings: Innovations, Quality, & Outcomes*, *4*(2), 211-215. https://doi.org/10.1016/j.mayocpiqo.2019.12.001

Muir-Cochrane, E., Grimmer, K., Gerace, A., Bastiampillai, T., & Oster, C. (2020). Prevalence of the use of chemical restraint in the management of challenging behaviors associated with adult mental health conditions: A meta-synthesis. *Journal of Psychiatric and Mental Health Nursing*, *27*(4), 425-445. https://doi.org/10.1111/jpm.12585

National Council of State Boards of Nursing. (2023). *Definition of nursing terms*. https://www.ncsbn.org/resources/nursing-terms.page

Nevels, M., Tinker, W., Zey, J. N., & Smith, T. (2020). Who is protecting healthcare professionals? Workplace violence & the occupational risk of providing care. *Professional Safety*, *65*(7), 39-43.

https://www.proquest.com/docview/2419751251/fulltextPDF/D3DEAAAB12DC4006PQ/1?accountid=12610

North Carolina Board of Nursing. (2023). *Registered Nurse.* https://www.ncbon.com/practice-registered-nurse#:~:text=PracticeRegistered%20Nurse,and%20related%20Administrative%20Code%20Rules.

Occupational Safety & Health Administration. (n.d.). *Workplace violence*. Retrieved on June 05, 2023, from https://www.osha.gov/workplace-violence#:~:text=What%20is%20workplace%20violence%3F,physical%20assaults%20and%20even%20homicide.

Ogboghodo, E. O., & Okojie, O. H. (2020). Workplace violence in the health sector: An assessment of prevalence and pattern. *European Journal of Public Health, 30,* 1-2. https://doi.org/10.1093/eurpub/ckaa166.1205

Orlando, I. J. P. (1961). *The dynamic nurse-patient relationship: Function, process, and principles.* National League for Nursing Practice.

Petiprin, A. (2023). *Orlando's nursing process discipline theory.* Nursing Theory. https://nursing-theory.org/theories-and-models/orlando-nursing-process-discipline-theory.php

Polit, D. F., & Beck, C. T. (2021). *Nursing research: Generating and assessing evidence for nursing practice* (11th ed.). Wolters Kluwer.

Roush, K. (2019). *A Nurse's step-by-step guide to writing a dissertation or scholarly project* (2nd ed.). Dustin Sullivan.

Sachdeva, S., Jamshed, N., Aggarwal, P., & Kashyap, S. R. (2019). Perception of workplace violence in the emergency department. *Journal of Emergencies, Trauma, and Shock, 12*(3), 179-184. https://doi.org/10.4103/JETS.JETS_81_18

Taghadosi, M., Valiee, S., & Aghajani, M. (2021). Nursing faculty's point of view regarding noncompliance with ethics in academic environments: A qualitative study. *BMC Nursing, 20*(1). https://doi.org/10.1186/s12912-021-00537-y

The Joint Commission. (18 June 2021). *R3 report: Requirement, rationale, reference.* https://www.jointcommission.org/standards/r3-report/r3-report-issue-38-national-patient-safety-goal-to-improve-health-care-equity/

The Joint Commission. (2023a). *Workplace violence prevention resources.* https://www.jointcommission.org/resources/patient-safety-topics/workplace-violence-prevention/

The Joint Commission. (2023b). *Who we are*. https://www.jointcommission.org/who-we-are/

United States Department of Labor. (n.d). *Occupational Safety and Health Administration*. Retrieved on June 03, 2023, from https://www.osha.gov/aboutosha

University of Mount Olive. (2018, November 15). *Institutional Review Board policies and procedures manual*. University of Mount Olive. https://storage.googleapis.com/zz-umo-o1spk6kr/media/edd4bf47-a460-4741-8fef-4c839ee1fabf/UMOIRBManual.pdf

www.ingramcontent.com/pod-product-compliance
Lightning Source LLC
LaVergne TN
LVHW041133150826
845673LV00007B/2297

* 9 7 8 3 3 8 4 2 5 9 5 5 4 *